Medical-Legal Disclaimer

This booklet is intended to provide general educational information for adult individuals looking to rule out craniocervical instability (CCI). It aims to offer guidance and improve patient understanding by outlining key considerations, such as how to choose a healthcare provider, what questions to ask, what to expect during diagnosis and treatment, and how to optimize self-care within the boundaries of established medical practice.

Although this booklet was not authored by a single leading specialist in the field, it was developed by a multidisciplinary team and the information presented is based on current clinical guidelines and the latest available peer-reviewed research at the time of publication. However, medical science is constantly evolving, and newer technologies or updated practices may not yet be reflected in this material.

This booklet does not provide medical advice. It is not intended to replace the personalized evaluation, diagnosis, or treatment recommendations of your licensed healthcare provider. The content should not in any way influence a patient's decisions, nor should it be considered a substitute for professional medical advice, nor does it establish a physician–patient relationship between the reader and any contributor to this publication. Each individual's medical condition is unique, and decisions regarding diagnosis, treatment, surgery, or rehabilitation should always be made in direct consultation with a qualified healthcare provider who is familiar with your complete medical history and current clinical status.

While every reasonable effort has been made to ensure the accuracy, clarity, and currency of the information provided, no guarantee can be made regarding its completeness, applicability, or relevance to every individual situation. The authors, contributors, medical researchers, medical editors, and the publisher disclaim any responsibility or liability for any loss, injury, or adverse outcomes that may result directly or indirectly from the use or application of the information contained in this publication.This resource is intended solely as a general guide for adults. Readers are encouraged to seek clarification from their healthcare providers about any specific medical questions or concerns.

A Patient's Guide to Craniocervical Instability Diagnosis
 ISBN 978-1-0698687-0-1

For permission requests, contact: Spine and Brain Advocate Publishing
www.spineandbrainadvocate.com Printed in the United States of America
Library and Archives Canada Cataloguing in Publication data available upon request.
Book Medical Editor: Dr. A. Bokhari, MD

A PATIENT'S GUIDE TO CRANIOCERVICAL INSTABILITY DIAGNOSIS

SPINEANDBRAINADVOCATE.COM

How to Use This Guide

This book is part of a three-book series created to support adult patients through every stage of their journey with craniocervical instability, from diagnosis, to fusion surgery, to long-term recovery.

You can read the book series straight through for the full picture, or jump directly to the book and chapters most relevant to you right now. Some patients start with Book 1 (Diagnosis), then move on to Book 2 (Surgery), and finally to Book 3 (Recovery). Others focus on just the book that matters most to them, returning to the other books if questions arise. Many people also find it useful to revisit certain sections over time, using the series as a guide at each stage of their journey.

While this guide provides medically reviewed information, it is not a substitute for medical advice. Always follow the instructions and recommendations of your physicians, surgeons, and healthcare team.

Table of Contents

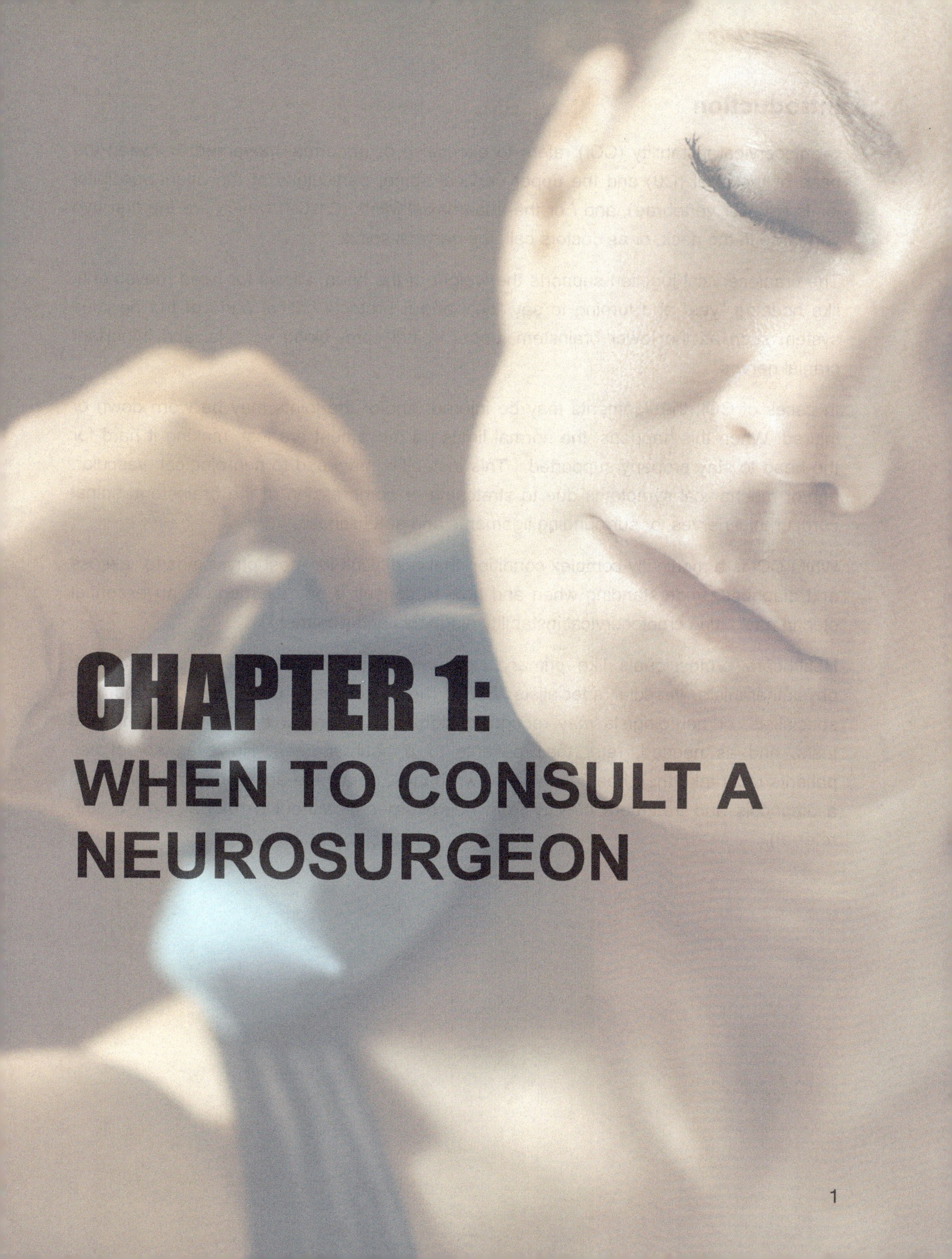

CHAPTER 1:
WHEN TO CONSULT A NEUROSURGEON

Introduction

Craniocervical instability (CCI) refers to excessive or abnormal movement between the base of the skull (C0) and the upper cervical spine, particularly at the atlanto-occipital joints (C0–C1 vertebrae), and / or the atlantoaxial joints (C1-C2), which are the first two vertebrae in the neck, or as doctors call, the cervical spine.

The craniocervical junction supports the weight of the head, allows for head movements like nodding "yes" and turning to say "no", and it protects critical parts of the nervous system such as the lower brainstem, upper spinal cord, blood vessels, and important cranial nerves.

In cases of CCI, the ligaments may be injured, and/or the joints may be worn down or injured. When this happens, the normal limits on movement are lost, making it hard for the head to stay properly supported. This instability may lead to neurological, vascular, and/or mechanical symptoms due to stretching or compression of the brainstem, spinal cord, cranial nerves, or surrounding ligaments and soft tissues.

While CCI is a medically complex condition that is difficult for most physicians to assess and diagnose, understanding when and how to consult a neurosurgeon is an essential step in navigating craniocervical instability diagnosis and treatment.

Healthcare professionals like primary care physicians, upper cervical chiropractors, physiotherapists, vascular specialists, ENTs, rheumatologists, Ehlers-danlos syndrome specialists, or neurologists *may* recognize signs of CCI, order adequate imaging and tests, and as needed, refer their patients to a neurosurgeon. However, sometimes patients must take their health into their own hands, obtain the appropriate imaging, and a diagnosis and treatment directly from neurosurgeons without a referral (i.e., a self-referral).

When CCI is diagnosed via clinical evaluation and imaging by a neurosurgeon, one possible treatment is craniocervical fusion (CCF) surgery. However, this is typically considered only after exhausting conservative treatment options or when symptoms are life-threatening or progressive. The decision to consult a neurosurgeon depends on key factors, such as:

- Symptom severity and frequency
- Radiological findings
- Failure of conservative treatments
- Degree of disability and quality of life
- Other patient-specific factors, such as:
    - Age
    - Overall health and other health conditions
    - Patient's wish for a peace of mind

This chapter offers a patient-focused guide to help individuals know when to seek a consultation with a neurosurgeon and how to prepare. It also explains why some neurosurgeons may overlook CCI unless it is caused by severe head and neck trauma, or well-known conditions like Down syndrome or rheumatoid arthritis, and what patients can do if that happens.

Symptoms Requiring Emergency Healthcare

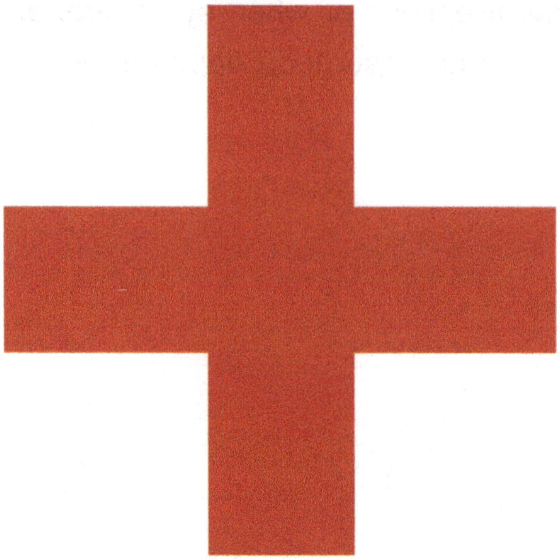

Before exploring when to consult a neurosurgeon, it's important to understand which symptoms require an urgent trip to the nearest emergency department. Certain symptoms can indicate serious, life-threatening conditions that demand immediate medical attention. In such cases, evaluation by an emergency room doctor is necessary.

Some symptoms that require urgent medical attention include:

- Severe difficulty breathing (*dyspnea*)
- Severe difficulty swallowing (*dysphagia*)
- Speech problems (*dysarthria*) i.e., weakness, paralysis, or lack of coordination of the muscles involved in speaking, which may affect clarity, pitch, volume, or speed of speech, making it difficult to speak clearly
- Loss of consciousness or fainting (*syncope*)
- Complete or partial paralysis
- Severe neck pain with numbness, tingling, or weakness in the limbs
- Imbalance and loss of coordination i.e., difficulty standing, walking, or coordinating hand–eye movements
- Persistent vomiting or nausea accompanied by a severe headache
- Vision loss or sudden blurred vision e.g., complete or partial blindness

- Sudden inability to control bowel movements or urination (*incontinence*), or difficulty urinating

- Severe chest pain or shortness of breath

- Severe headache with vision changes e.g., visual disturbances, blurred vision, or double vision

- Drop attacks or loss of muscle control i.e., sudden, unexplained weakness or collapse without loss of consciousness

- Severe or uncontrolled tremors affecting the arms, legs, or entire body

- Sudden loss of sensation or weakness in one or more limbs

- Severe dizziness or vertigo that makes it difficult to stand or maintain balance

Understand what symptoms require an urgent trip to the nearest emergency department.

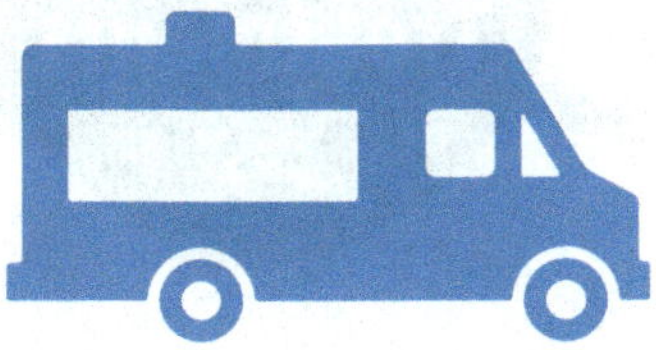

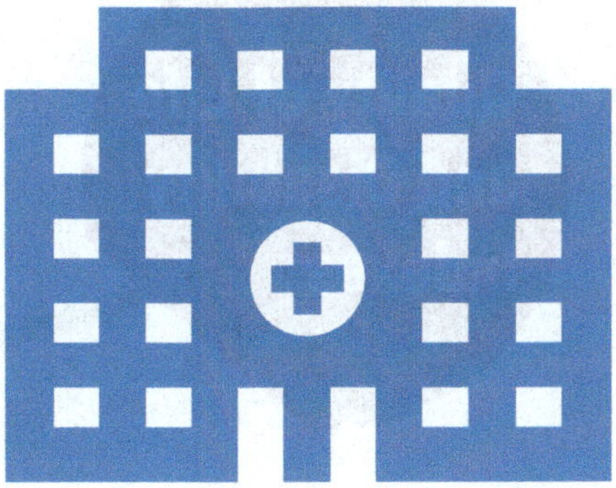

Neurosurgical Consultation Decision Framework

Patients advocating for their healthcare is an essential part of managing one's own health and well-being. Consulting a neurosurgeon can be a critical decision that is based on key criteria such as a patient's symptoms, diagnostic findings, and the overall impact of the condition on their quality of life.

The following proposed neurosurgical consultation decision framework is a helpful tool to assist patients and their caregivers in determining whether and when to seek a neurosurgeon's input.

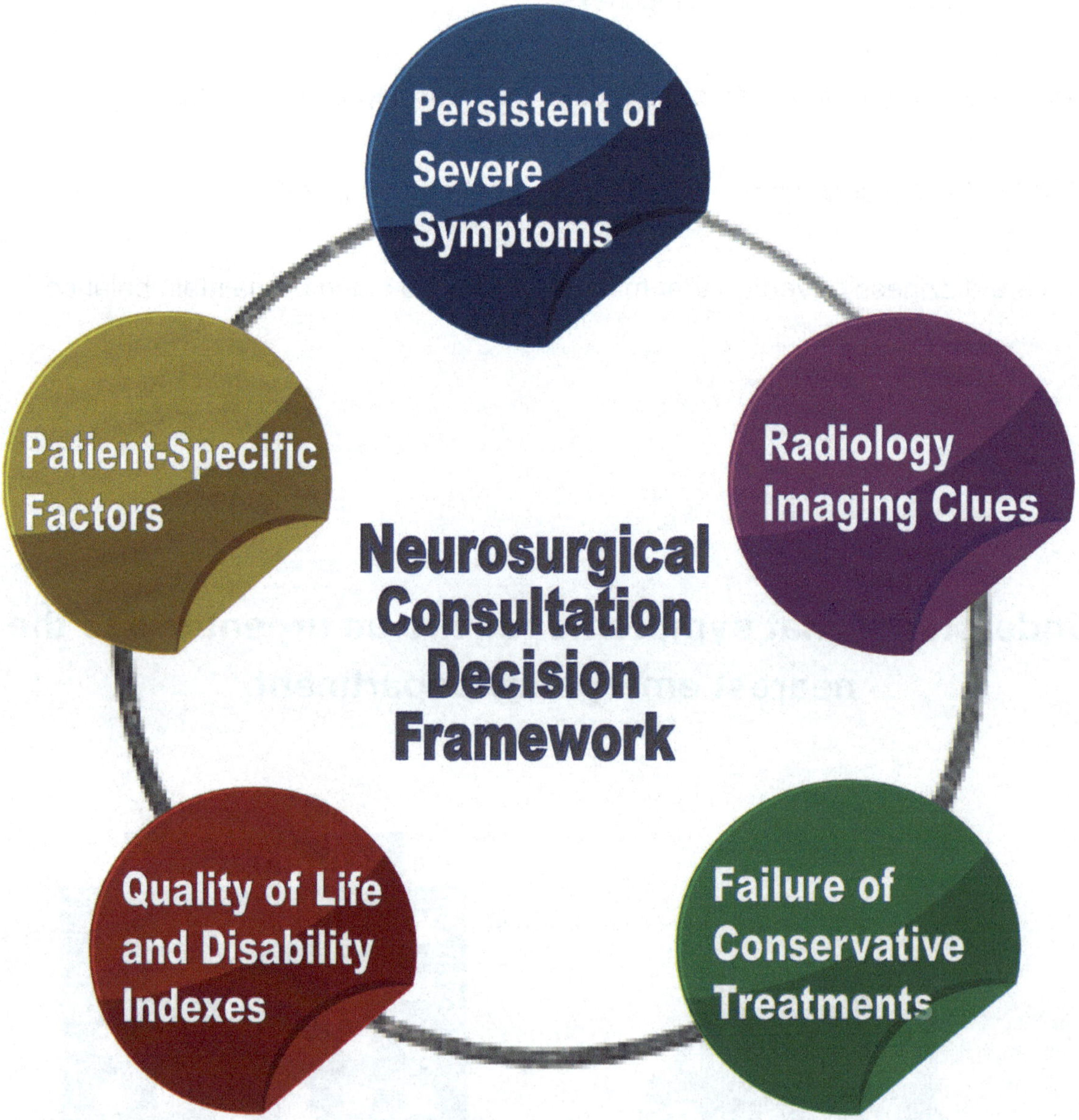

Key Decision Factor #1 - Persistent or Severe Symptoms

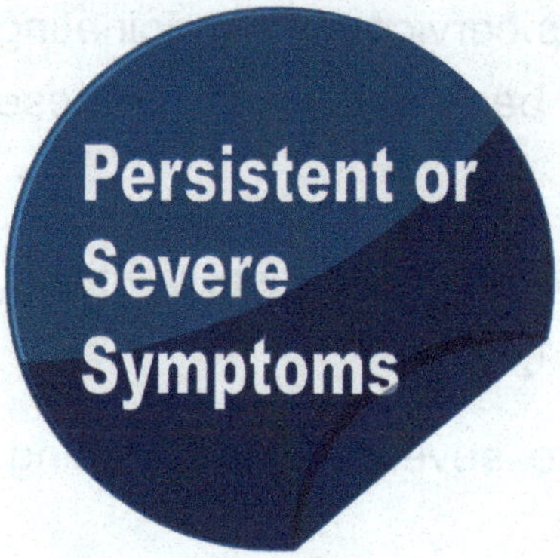

The following outlines common symptom-based categories of craniocervical instability, along with their subtypes or specific symptom examples. Patients seeking diagnosis and treatment would benefit from documenting a summary list of their symptoms and subtypes, listing those with the highest severity and frequency at the top of the list, and those with the least severity and frequency at the bottom, using the medical severity and frequency scales noted in this chapter.

Patients should try to keep this document to a maximum of one page, including any notes on the date and event leading to the onset of these symptoms, if applicable (e.g., trauma onset, viral onset, or unknown onset).

Common Symptoms

1. ⚡ **Pain Symptoms**

    - **Neck Pain:** Pain at the base of the skull and neck that can radiate (i.e., spread) to the jaw, shoulders, and upper back. The pain may worsen with movement or certain head positions. This is the most common manifestation, often spreading to the arms and may be accompanied by occipital headache radiating to the back of the skull or widespread pain (i.e., fibromyalgia).
    - **Heavy Head Sensation:** A "bobblehead" feeling, as if the head is too heavy for the neck to support, causing difficulty being upright for long periods of time.
    - **Muscle Tightness:** Tightness, stiffness, and trigger points in the muscles around the neck, shoulder, chest, and upper back. This can feel like discomfort when moving or turning the head.
    - **Facial Pain:** Pain in the face, especially around the eyes, temples, or jaw.
    - **Tenderness at the base of the skull:** Pain localized to the base of the skull.

2. 👤 **Headache Symptoms**

- **Chronic Headaches:** Persistent headaches, often felt as cervicogenic (originating from the neck) or occipital headaches (coming from the back of the head). These may be worsened by certain movements or positions.
- **Chronic Migraines:** Intense headaches, often accompanied by nausea, vomiting, and sensitivity to light and sound, often cervicogenic in origin.
- **Positional Headaches:** Headaches that become more severe when standing, sitting up, or changing positions.
- **Pressure Headaches:** Sensation of pressure around the head, sometimes felt behind one or both eyes.
- **Occipital Headaches:** Pain that begins at the back of the head, often radiating to the neck and sometimes the face.

3. 👁 **Vision Symptoms**

- **Blurred Vision:** Difficulty seeing clearly or sudden changes in vision, such as intermittent blurriness, or experiencing visual disturbances.
- **Visual Snow:** The perception of "static" or "snow" in the visual field, similar to a TV signal with interference.
- **Floaters:** Small, moving specks or shapes in the field of vision.
- **Temporary Loss of Vision:** Sudden or transient temporary loss of part or all of the field of vision.
- **Light Sensitivity:** Sensitivity or intolerance to light or difficulty tolerating bright environments, making it difficult to see in lit environments.
- **Double Vision (Diplopia):** Seeing two images of a single object.
- **Irregular Eye Movements:** Jerky, uncoordinated eye movements, especially in response to head motion.
- **Involuntary eye movements (Nystagmus):** When the eyes make involuntary, repetitive movements.

4. 👂 **Ear & Hearing Symptoms**

- **Ear Pressure:** Pain with temporary hearing loss and a feeling of fullness or pressure in the ears.
- **Tinnitus:** Ringing, buzzing, or hissing sounds in the ears, which may be constant or intermittent.
- **Pulsatile Tinnitus:** Ringing or buzzing in time with the heartbeat.
- **Positional Tinnitus:** Tinnitus that changes with head position.
- **Vertigo:** A sensation of spinning or dizziness, as if the room is moving.

5. 📈 **Cardiovascular and Autonomic Symptoms**

- **Postural Orthostatic Tachycardia Syndrome (POTS):** A condition where the heart rate increases significantly, by at least 30 beats per minute, within 10 minutes of standing, causing dizziness, lightheadedness, and sometimes fainting.
- **Bradycardia:** Slow heart rate slower than 60 beats per minute, that can cause fatigue, dizziness, or fainting spells.
- **Tachycardia:** Rapid heart rate exceeding 100 beats per minute at rest, often felt as heart palpitations.
- **Heat Intolerance:** Difficulty tolerating heat and may involve excessive sweating. An exaggerated physiological response to heat exposure including a rise in core body temperature, heart rate and sometimes changes blood pressure.
- **Orthostatic Hypotension:** A sudden drop in blood pressure (specifically when systolic blood pressure drops by at least 20 mmHg or diastolic blood pressure drops by at least 10 mmHg within 2 to 3 minutes upon standing, often leading to dizziness, fainting, or lightheadedness.

6. Throat, Voice and Swallowing Symptoms

- **Difficulty Swallowing (Dysphagia):** Trouble swallowing food, liquids, or even saliva.
- **Reduced Gag Reflex:** A diminished or reduced gag reflex, which can make swallowing more difficult and increase the risk of choking or something swallowed goes down the wrong way (aspiration).
- **Hoarseness:** A raspy or weak voice and can be caused by irritation, inflammation, vocal cord injury, or nerve issues.
- **Voice Changes:** Difficulty speaking clearly or projecting voice.

7. Gastrointestinal (GI) Symptoms

- **Nausea and Vomiting:** Chronic nausea, often leading to vomiting.
- **Bloating:** A sensation of fullness or swelling in the abdomen, often associated with delayed gastric emptying.
- **Constipation:** Difficulty passing stools, or infrequent bowel movements.
- **Diarrhea:** Frequent, loose stools.
- **Heartburn and Reflux:** Gastroesophageal reflux disease (GERD), where stomach acid backs up into the esophagus, causing discomfort or a burning sensation in the chest.
- **Abdominal Pain:** Cramping or discomfort in the abdomen.
- **Delayed gastric emptying (gastroparesis):** When the stomach empties food into the small intestine slower than normal.
- **Incontinence:** Loss of control over bowel (fecal incontinence) or bladder (urinary incontinence) functions. While typically categorized separately from gastrointestinal symptoms, it is relevant in discussions of pelvic floor or autonomic dysfunction.

8. 🧠 **Cognitive and Psychological Symptoms**

- **Brain Fog:** Difficulty thinking clearly, concentrating, or processing information. This can feel like mental cloudiness or sluggishness.
- **Memory Problems:** Issues with short-term memory, such as forgetting names, appointments, or where items are placed.
- **Loss of Words:** Difficulty recalling words, terms, or names, often occurring during conversations.
- **Anxiety and Panic Attacks:** Feelings of intense anxiety, panic or flight or flight.
- **Mood Swings:** Sudden changes in mood, including increased irritability or depression.

9. 🛌 **Sleep Issues and Chronic Fatigue Symptoms**

- **Chronic Fatigue:** Severe, persistent fatigue that lasts for at least six months and is not substantially relieved by rest.
- **Post-exertional malaise (PEM):** A worsening of symptoms after minimal physical or mental exertion.
- **Insomnia:** Difficulty falling asleep or staying asleep.
- **Sleep Apnea:** Repeated interruptions of breathing during sleep. There are two main types:
    - Obstructive Sleep Apnea (OSA): Caused by physical blockage of the airway.
    - Central Sleep Apnea (CSA): Caused by the brain's failure to send proper signals to the muscles that control breathing.
    - Mixed sleep apnea involves features of both.

💡 **Remember**, the above listed symptoms do not necessarily determine CCI, as they can be caused by a variety of diseases or disorders. A proper diagnosis requires a thorough evaluation by a neurosurgeon, ideally one that specializes in craniocervical instability.

Assessing Symptoms Using Scales

Medical symptom assessment scales are tools that are used to help patients and physicians turn subjective symptom experiences into measurable information by rating symptom disruptiveness, intensity, and frequency. Patient's are encouraged to discuss locally-utilized symptom assessment scales with their healthcare provider. They can benefit from knowing about and using symptom scales to help guide productive discussions around the patient's health. There are many medical symptom assessment scales utilized around the world, however only the following symptom scales will be briefly reviewed in this chapter:

1. The **Likert scale** to track how much symptoms interfere with daily life.
2. A **symptom frequency scale** to track how often symptoms occur within a specific time period.
3. A **numbered pain intensity scale** to monitor pain severity.

Symptom assessment scales help make communication clearer, supports diagnosis, and helps track how symptoms change over time. By showing how much symptoms interfere with daily life, these tools also guide treatment decisions and the need for specialist care.

1. Likert Scale for Disruptiveness or Burden of Symptoms

The Likert Scale is a 5-point scale (or sometimes a 7-point scale) tool used to rate how much a symptom *interferes* with a patient's daily life. It helps both patients and healthcare providers communicate the real-life impact of symptoms, such as how much they limit work, sleep, mobility, or self-care. By assigning a level from "None" to "Very Severe," the scale offers a structured way to track changes over time and guide treatment decisions, including when to consider specialist care, like neurosurgery.

Here is the Likert Scale:

1. **None:** No symptoms or issues present.
2. **Mild:** Symptoms are noticeable but do not significantly impact daily activities.
3. **Moderate:** Symptoms are clearly present and may cause some discomfort or affect daily functioning.
4. **Severe:** Symptoms are intense and noticeably interfere with daily tasks and quality of life.
5. **Very Severe:** Symptoms are extremely intense and debilitating, severely affecting all aspects of life.

2. Assessing Frequency of Symptoms

Frequency scales are used to assess how *often* a symptom *occurs* within a certain time frame. They help identify symptom patterns and evaluate responses to treatment. One commonly used example of the numeric frequency scale is as follows:

Numeric Frequency Scale for Symptom Persistence:

0 = Never

1 = Rarely (less than once a week)

5 = Occasionally (once a week or more)

10 = Constantly (occur almost daily, but not all day long without stopping)

3. Numeric Pain Intensity Scale

The pain scale categorizes pain into levels from 0 to 10, which describe the *intensity* of the pain. These levels are grouped together into mild, moderate, and severe pain. Here's how it breaks down:

"0" is no pain.

Mild Pain (1 to 3)

- Level 1: Barely noticeable and easily ignored.
- Level 2: Mildly annoying.
- Level 3: Distracting, but the patient can learn to adapt to it.

Moderate Pain (4 to 6)

- Level 4: Able to push pain aside for periods while involved in a task, but it is still very distracting.

- Level 5: Pain can't be ignored for more than a few minutes, but the patient can be tolerated with effort.
- Level 6: Pain may make it hard for the patient to concentrate on regular tasks.

Severe Pain (7 to 10)

- Level 7: Pain demands a patient's attention and keeps them from performing tasks. It may interfere with sleep.
- Level 8: Pain is intense, limiting physical activity and making conversation difficult.
- Level 9: Patient is unable to converse and may just be moaning or crying.
- Level 10: Pain leaves the patient bedridden or even delirious.

Frequency Scale to Assess How Often a Symptom Occurs

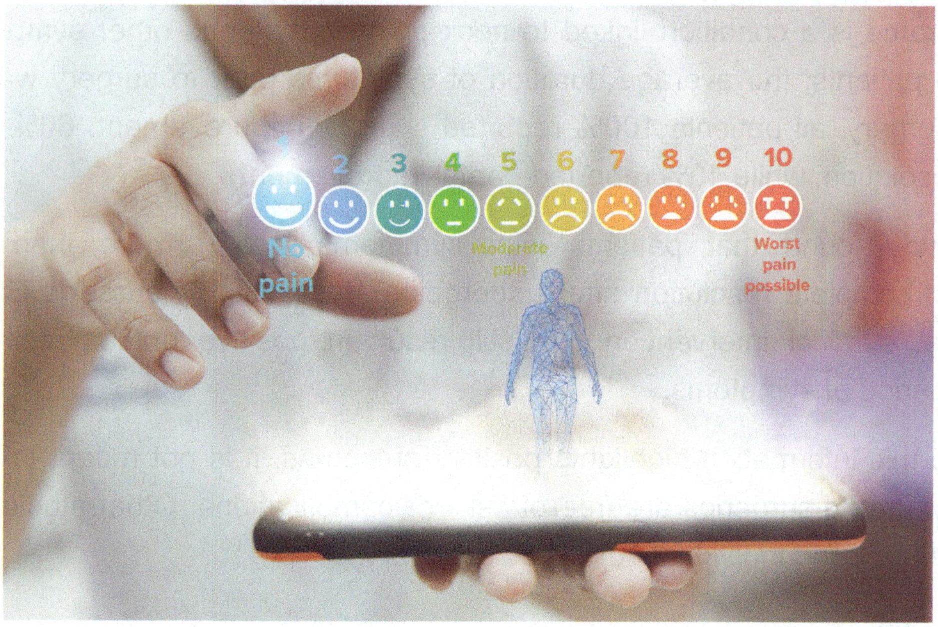

Symptom Severity and the Impact of Early Surgical Intervention

For patients dealing with CCI, understanding whether surgery can improve their symptoms, prevent further complications, or enhance their overall well-being is crucial for making informed treatment decisions. Research on CCI symptom severity and *early* surgical intervention is limited, however, existing studies on other neck related conditions emphasize that timely surgery can significantly improve health-related quality of life for patients with neurological symptoms linked to cervical spine (neck issues).

Evidence from broader spine surgery literature suggests that the timing of surgery is a key factor in recovery. When deemed appropriate, earlier surgical intervention is generally associated with improved outcomes. According to some studies, delays in intervention are linked to poorer outcomes, while early surgical treatment is generally associated with better recovery and enhanced quality of life. The following studies demonstrate how symptom severity and duration influence recovery outcomes across different surgical procedures:

Eagle Syndrome Study

Eagle syndrome is a condition linked to neck pain and various other symptoms. In one study of 56 patients, the average duration of symptoms prior to surgery was 4.1 years. Following surgery, all patients 100% reported symptom improvement: 60% experienced complete resolution, while 40% reported partial improvement.

Another study found that patients with symptoms lasting more than 12 months experienced complete resolution after undergoing styloidectomy surgery. These findings suggest that surgical intervention can still result in positive outcomes, even after a prolonged period of symptoms.

Note: While this information highlights positive outcomes, it is not meant to suggest that all Eagle syndrome surgeries are free of risks or complications. Other studies report less favorable results, and individual outcomes may vary.

Cervical Radiculopathy Study

Cervical radiculopathy, or a pinched nerve in the neck, can usually improve within 4 to 8 weeks with rest, physical therapy, and medication. If symptoms persist, surgery may be necessary. When performed early, typically within 8 weeks, it may improve recovery and reduce healthcare costs. Research also shows that delaying surgery beyond two years can lead to poorer outcomes, while surgery performed within six months generally results in better health and quality of life.

Study on Brain and Neck Cancer Patients with Swallowing & Vision Problems

A study on head and neck cancer patients showed that difficulty swallowing (dysphagia) and low health-related quality of life (HRQoL) scores before surgery can lead to longer hospital stays and higher readmission rates after surgery. This study suggests that having symptoms for a long time before surgery can make recovery harder and affect overall well-being. This study also highlights that by assessing patient-reported outcomes and quality of life (QOL) before surgery, doctors can identify patients who may be at risk for longer hospital stays and more health care needs after leaving the hospital. Early intervention and careful monitoring of symptoms may help improve recovery and reduce complications.

Cervical Myelopathy Study

A study involving 98 patients who underwent posterior cervical decompression and fusion (PCDF) for cervical myelopathy (a condition where the spinal cord in the neck gets compressed) found that those with symptoms lasting more than 2 years showed significantly less improvement in myelopathy scores (mJOA) and neck disability index (NDI) postoperatively.

In contrast, patients with symptoms lasting less than 6 months demonstrated substantial improvements in these measures.

Key Takeaways on When to Consider Surgery

When conservative treatments for neurological symptoms related to cervical spine conditions fail, consulting a neurosurgeon is an important step. Patients who do not experience improvement in neurological symptoms after several months of treatments such as physical therapy, medications, or injections may benefit from a surgical evaluation.

Although there is no exact timeline, many neurosurgeons suggest seeking an opinion after about 6 months of unsuccessful conservative treatment, depending on the severity and urgency of the symptoms.

In patients with severe neurological symptoms related to neck related issues, delaying surgery for too long, especially beyond two years, may lead to less favorable outcomes, while early intervention may result in better recovery and improved health-related quality of life (HRQoL). This is particularly true in conditions such as cervical radiculopathy and cervical myelopathy, where symptoms that persist for longer periods can complicate recovery.

Early diagnosis and treatment are crucial for preventing complications, reducing the risk of further neurological damage, and optimizing post-surgical quality of life.

Specialists can help determine whether surgery is the best option, based on the patient's specific condition and needs, potentially improving the chances of a successful recovery.

Early Diagnosis and Treatment Matters.

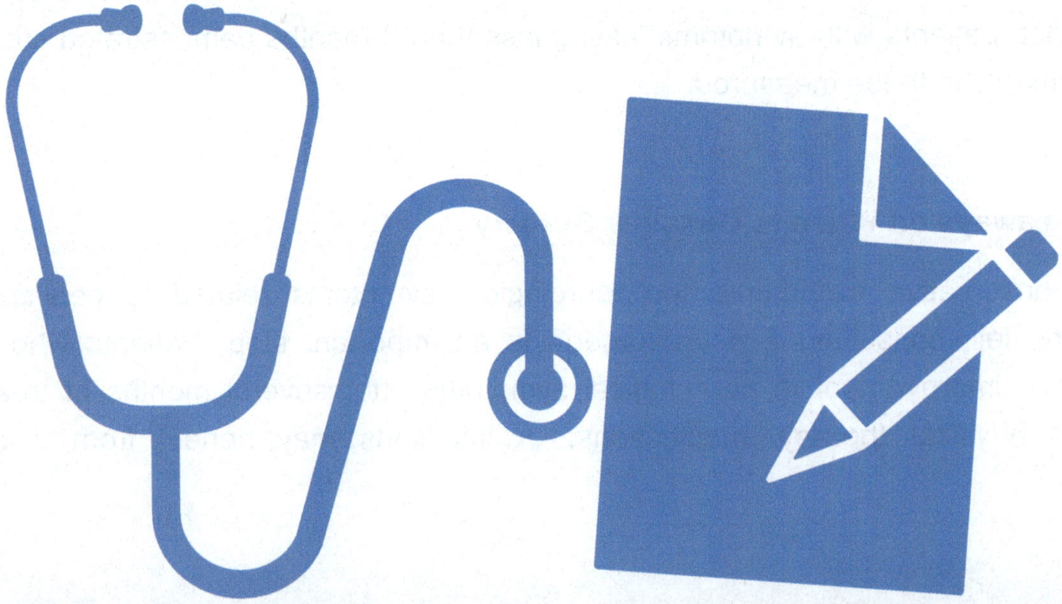

Neurological Symptoms: An Important Consideration

Patients with CCI may experience a variety of neurological symptoms affecting sensation, movement, speech, and cognitive function. Recognizing these symptoms early, no matter their frequency, and reporting them immediately to a healthcare provider can be crucial in guiding diagnosis and treatment decisions.

Common neurological signs include:

- ☐ Sensations of numbness, tingling, or "pins and needles" in the arms, hands, or legs.
- ☐ A feeling of weakness in the arms, hands, or legs making it difficult to hold objects, walk, or stand without support.
- ☐ Impaired coordination such as difficulty with fine motor skills, or frequent dropping of objects.
- ☐ Paralysis
- ☐ Walking disturbances
- ☐ Involuntary shaking or tremors, which can affect the hands, arms, or legs.
- ☐ Dystonic Seizures (uncontrolled muscle contractions leading to abnormal, repetitive twisting movements, particularly in the limbs or neck).
- ☐ Slurred or unclear speech due to muscle control problems.
- ☐ Difficulty swallowing food, liquids, or saliva.
- ☐ Changes in voice quality, often becoming raspy or strained.
- ☐ Difficulty controlling bowel or bladder function
- ☐ Changes in memory, thinking, or mood

Tracking Symptoms

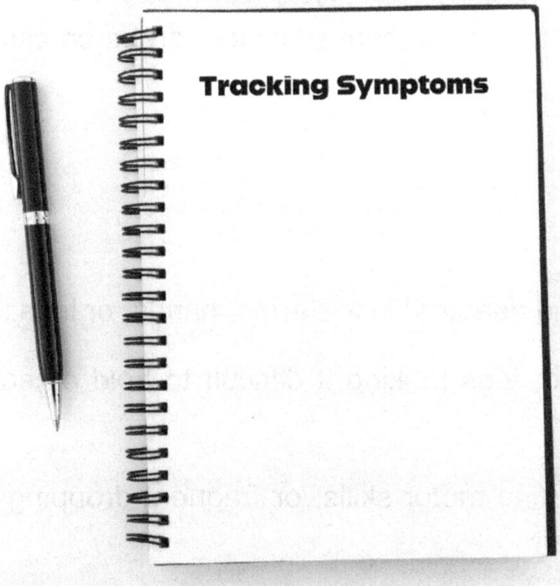

The recording of symptoms is a key factor in assessing how a condition impacts a patient's daily life and overall well-being. These factors often guide decisions about diagnosis, treatment, and whether to refer a patient to specialist care. It's important that patients track their symptoms to present to their healthcare team. Some specialists appreciate a great level of detail such as symptom triggers, and organization of top concerning symptoms first, as this helps guide their assessment approach.

Physicians may ask patients to complete symptom questionnaires to assess these aspects. Patients can also take the initiative to fill out relevant questionnaires or tracking tools and bring them to medical appointments. These can support more productive, focused discussions with healthcare teams.

Because symptoms can change over time, it's important for patients to record and update their symptoms regularly. This may include:

- Noting symptom severity and frequency, and highlighting neurological symptoms
- Recording the context of symptom episodes (e.g., activity at onset, duration, triggers, certain head positions).
- Listing symptoms in order of severity or impact

Unfortunately, there is currently no single, universally accepted neurosurgical assessment tool for CCI or CCJ disorders. Each neurosurgeon may use different evaluation methods and criteria. This makes clear, organized symptom tracking especially important for patients seeking a diagnosis or second opinion.

Patients should create a running list of symptoms starting with those that are most severe and most frequent. Include severity and frequency scores, the date of onset, and if known, what may have triggered the symptom (e.g., an injury, illness, or unknown cause). This list should be brought to all relevant medical appointments and updated over time. It can also help the patient manage his or her symptoms by managing or avoiding the contexts that bring on or exacerbate symptoms.

Patient Symptom Tracking Worksheet Sample

Patients seeking a diagnosis or treatment should keep a simple, up-to-date list of their symptoms. This list should start with the most severe and frequent symptoms, using the rating scales provided in this chapter. It should also include the date symptoms began and any known cause, such as an injury or illness.

A summary document should be kept to one page, stored in a safe place, and clearly dated. Keeping this record current helps healthcare providers better understand the patient's condition and how it is progressing.

Patients who have had craniocervical fusion or other surgeries should track their symptoms before their follow-up appointments, as well as bring the summary document to their physiotherapy and other relevant medical appointments.

SYMPTOM TRACKING WORKSHEET SAMPLE

Name:	Date:		Date:		Date:	
LIST OF SYMPTOMS	Severity	Frequency	Severity	Frequency	Severity	Frequency
PAIN SYMPTOMS						
Neck Pain						
Heavy Head Sensations						
Muscle Tightness						
Facial Pain						
Tenderness at Base of Skull						
HEADACHE SYMPTOMS						
Chronic Headaches						
Chronic Migraines						
Positional Headaches						
Pressure Headaches						
Occipital Headaches						
VISION SYMPTOMS						

Blurred Vision						
Visual Snow						
Floaters						
Light Sensitivity						
Loss of / Double Vision						
Involuntary eye movements						
EAR AND HEARING SYMPTOMS						
Hearing loss or ear fullness or pressure in / area of the ears						
Tinnitus						
Pulsatile Tinnitus						
Positional Tinnitus						
Vertigo						
CARDIOVASCULAR AND AUTONOMIC SYMPTOMS						
POTS						
Bradycardia						
Tachycardia						
Heat Intolerance						
Orthostatic Hypotension						
THROAT, VOICE & SWALLOWING SYMPTOMS						
Difficulty Swallowing						
Reduced Gag Reflex						
Hoarseness						
Voice Changes						
GASTROINTESTINAL SYMPTOMS						
Nausea and Vomiting						

Bloating						
Constipation						
Diarrhea						
Heartburn and Reflux						
Abdominal Pain						
Delayed gastric emptying and / or incontinence						
COGNITIVE & PSYCHOLOGICAL SYMPTOMS						
Brain Fog						
Memory Problems						
Loss of Words						
Anxiety						
Panic Attacks						
Mood Swings						
Depression						
SLEEP ISSUES AND CHRONIC FATIGUE SYMPTOMS						
Chronic debilitating fatigue						
Post-exertional malaise (PEM)						
Insomnia						
Sleep Apnea						
Other:						
Other:						
Other:						

Key Decision Factor #2 - Radiology Measurements & Clues

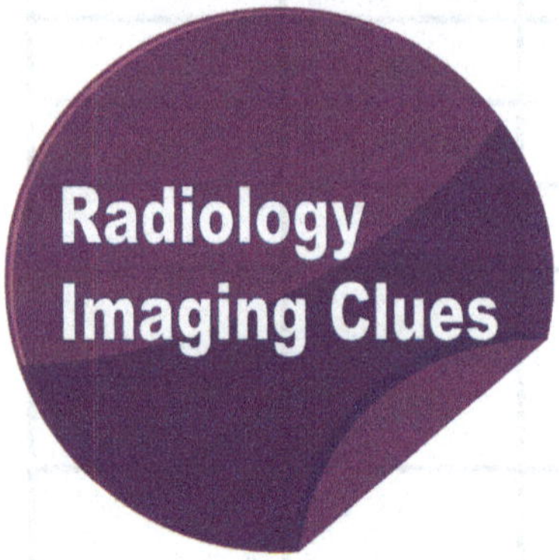

Medical imaging is a key tool in helping to diagnose CCI and related conditions. Because the area between the base of the skull and the upper spine is highly complex, doctors rely on advanced imaging to help detect problems.

This includes dynamic MRI and CT scan radiology studies, which involve a series of head and neck positions such as neutral, flexion (chin to chest), extension (looking up), and rotation (turning the head left and right), ideally in upright position (performed while standing or sitting position); as opposed to laying down (supine) imaging studies.

These medical imaging tests help show how the bones, soft tissues, blood flow, and cerebrospinal fluid (CSF) are functioning. They can also reveal abnormal motion or malalignment in this critical area. However, having the right imaging is only part of the process.

The quality of the imaging is important too, and the imaging studies must be interpreted by specialists with advanced training. These specialists include neuroradiologists, who focus on the brain, head, neck, and spine and neurosurgeons, particularly those specializing in the craniocervical junction (CCJ) / base of skull.

Some of these experts can detect subtle findings or abnormalities and CCI. While these may not confirm a problem on their own, they could suggest an issue, especially when symptoms are present. This is why a scan may be reported as “normal” by a general radiologist, even when a potential problem exists.

Expert interpretation is essential for an accurate diagnosis. Physicians should ensure that imaging requests include clear instructions to perform scans of the cervical spine and craniocervical junction in upright, dynamic positions, whenever possible. It is also important that the radiologist interpreting the scans has specific experience with CCI.

In some cases, patients may need to proactively seek out appropriate specialists themselves. Patients may also consider using third-party radiology opinion services, which offer remote reviews of existing imaging. These services can provide fast and convenient second opinions; however, it is essential to confirm that the radiologists involved are experienced in reporting on CCI and its common comorbidities.

High Radiology Error Rates

Radiology mistakes are more common than most people think, and can lead to serious consequences such as delayed diagnoses, incorrect treatment, or long-term health problems. Studies show that reported error rates in radiology can range from roughly 20% to 40%. This means that in some cases, “normal” imaging reports may not be accurate.

These errors can happen at many stages:

- If the ordering doctor doesn’t clearly state the concerns or differential diagnoses, such as ruling out issues related to the CCJ, the radiologist may not focus on the right areas.
- Technologists might take images from the wrong angles, use poor technique or accept poor quality images.
- The radiologist reading the images may not have the specialized knowledge needed to complete an accurate report, or the healthcare system does not acknowledge the conditions being investigated.

It’s important to make sure your imaging is done correctly so that your diagnosis is accurate. This means three things:

1) get the right type of imaging ordered for the medical condition(s) / symptoms to be assessed

2) at the imaging center, double-check that the technician and radiologist will follow the order exactly and not take shortcuts, and

3) make sure the radiology report fully evaluates for craniocervical instability (CCI). If there's any doubt, consider getting a second opinion from a specialist.

In cases where CCI is suspected, reducing imaging errors leads to more accurate diagnoses, faster and safer treatment, fewer unnecessary procedures, and better long-term outcomes for patients. Being aware that imaging errors can occur is important, and having scans for CCI and its comorbidities interpreted by CCI experts is critical to ensuring an accurate diagnosis and appropriate care.

Note: Many patients struggle to access specialists who understand CCI, Eagle syndrome and tethered cord syndrome. Due to delays in referrals or a lack of physician awareness, patients frequently advocate for their own healthcare by obtaining their own images, and seeking second radiology and neurosurgical opinions.

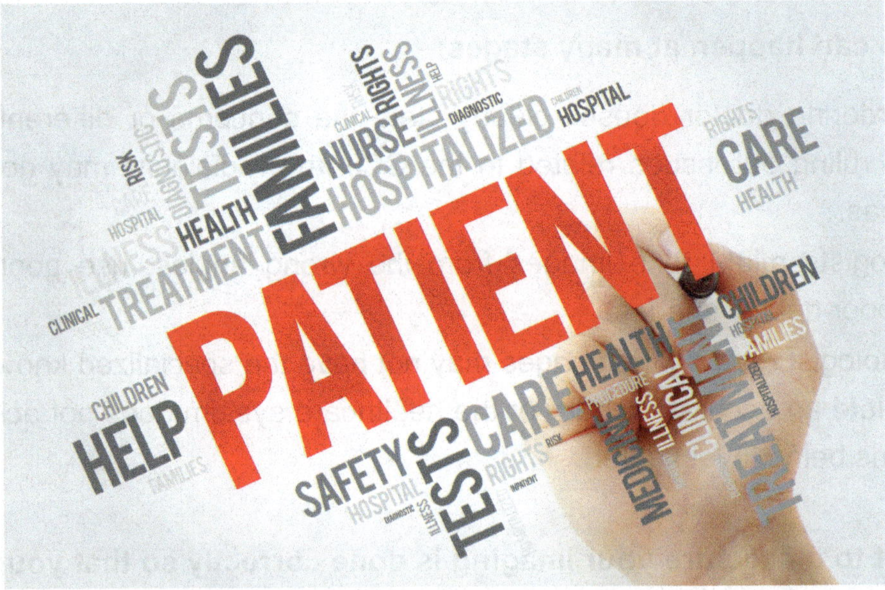

Key Diagnostic Imaging for Assessing Craniocervical Junction

The following are general radiology imaging guidelines to check for craniocervical instability. It's important to understand that a single imaging study is usually not enough to thoroughly investigate the structural and mechanical issues that may be causing a patients symptoms.

1. Dynamic 3D Upright Cone Beam CT (uCBCT) or **3D CT (Computed Tomography) scan** in neck positions of neutral, flexion, extension (and if possible, rotation left and right) are the **gold standard** for evaluating craniocervical instability. Both modalities allow the measuring the *bony structures* of the CCJ, cervical spine, base of the skull, and assessing other key anatomy such as the C1 transverse processes and styloid processes. This study helps *infer* laxity or injury of the ligaments based on the degree or amount of movement rather than appearance alone.

CT scans are excellent for showing fine details of the bones, especially with 0.75 mm to *maximum of 1 mm* imaging slices and reformatting in both the coronal and sagittal planes provides 3D images with detailed visualization of the bony relationships and congruency of the craniocervical junction.

The uCBCT generally uses less radiation compared to traditional CT scans, however it provides slightly less quality images than CT scans. uCBCTs are completed with the patient standing in upright position, which helps visualize how the head and neck can be affected by gravity, which is advantageous over the CT scans. uCBCTs are available in some upper cervical chiropractor's offices, typically NUCCA and Blair practitioners. (nucca.org / blairchiropractic.com)

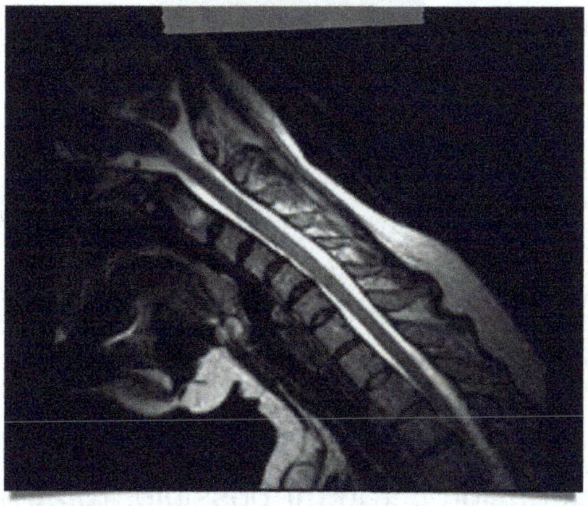

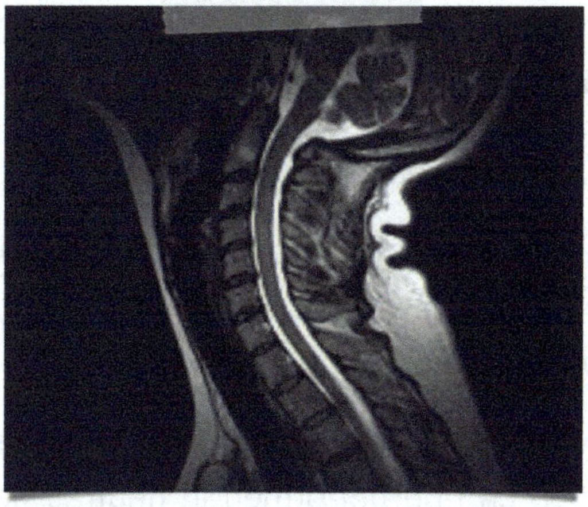

MRI Cervical Spine and Craniocervical Junction in Flexion-Extension Positions

2. Dynamic upright MRI (uMRI) Cervical Spine and Craniocervical Junction in neutral, flexion and extension positions is the gold standard for assessing the soft tissues of the CCJ and cervical spine in different positions, with the weight of gravity, however, it is not always locally accessible.

An alternative to the dynamic uMRI is the supine (lying down) MRI Cervical Spine and Craniocervical Junction in neutral position which used to examine *soft tissues* (i.e. the spinal cord and ligaments) for injuries, degenerative conditions, and other abnormalities including CCI, however, doctors writing the requisition should write "include a high-resolution assessment of brainstem, alar and transverse ligaments, and other soft tissues for injuries") as this component is considered a specialized assessment and would not be included in a standard MRI of the cervical spine. Ideally the radiologist will use a 3T MRI, or alternatively a 1.5T MRI with the use of a dedicated head/neck coil with coverages down to C2, MPR (multiple planes), thin-slice protocol, ideally in small voxel size and a proton-density weighted sequence or equivalent high-resolution sequence.

3. MRI Brain helps to assess the brain's structures and tissues. This study helps to rule out chiari malformation, differential diagnosis, and assess patterns of brain changes caused by neurodegeneration, since neurodegenerative disorders and CCI have significant symptom overlap.

Together, these imaging studies compliment each other and provide a more wholistic examination to rule out craniocervical instability and abnormalities of the craniocervical junction.

What To Do When A Dynamic 3D CT Scan or A Dynamic 3D uCBCT Are Not Available

Viable alternatives include:

- A Dynamic X-Ray Series of Cervical Spine and Craniocervical Junction in positions of neutral, flexion, extension (and if possible, rotation left and right and lateral side bending (ear to shoulder) right and left.

-A dynamic digital radiography (DDR) X-ray movie in radiology DICOM format (by Konica Minolta's) can be performed in neutral, flexion, extension (and if possible, rotation left and right and lateral side bending (ear to shoulder) right and left. The DICOM format allows radiologists to measure the instability versus other X-ray movie formats like DMX are not measurable in radiology standards.

However, although X-rays are more affordable and accessible, they produce lower quality images, which means there's a higher chance of missing something important.

Be Mindful to Avoid Imaging Issues

Complete Imaging Requisition

Accurate diagnostic imaging begins with a complete requisition. As discussed earlier in the section on high radiology error rates, one of the most common problems is that requisition forms are submitted with incomplete or vague information. This can prevent the radiology team from performing the correct imaging protocol or reporting results thoroughly.

Many patients and families make significant financial and personal sacrifices to obtain advanced imaging, sometimes even paying out of pocket, only to discover later that the requisition was inadequate. By working with their healthcare provider to ensure that the requisition is filled out in detail, patients and caregivers can play an active role in reducing errors and improving the quality of their diagnostic studies.

Safety / Contraindications

Patients must provide information to the radiologist, ideally well in advance of the appointment, about contrast allergies or reactions, abnormal renal function, implanted devices, and if they are pregnant. It helps the radiologist tailor the right approach and avoid complications.

Patients Can Help Prevent Imaging Errors

As also noted in the section on radiology error rates, problems can arise when imaging clinics modify or override a requisition without the ordering provider's input, or when the equipment available at the clinic cannot support the requested protocols. Patients and caregivers can reduce the risk of errors by confirming in advance that the clinic has the capability to perform the requested imaging and, at the time of the appointment, by speaking with the technologist or radiologist to ensure the study is carried out as ordered and that all necessary information is available to fulfill the requisition.

Radiology-Based Assessment of the Craniocervical Junction

Several key radiological measurements are used to evaluate CCI. These measurements help provide an objective assessment of the CCJ, potentially opening doors to specialist appointments and guide treatment decisions, ensuring appropriate care for individuals experiencing abnormalities and instability at the CCJ.

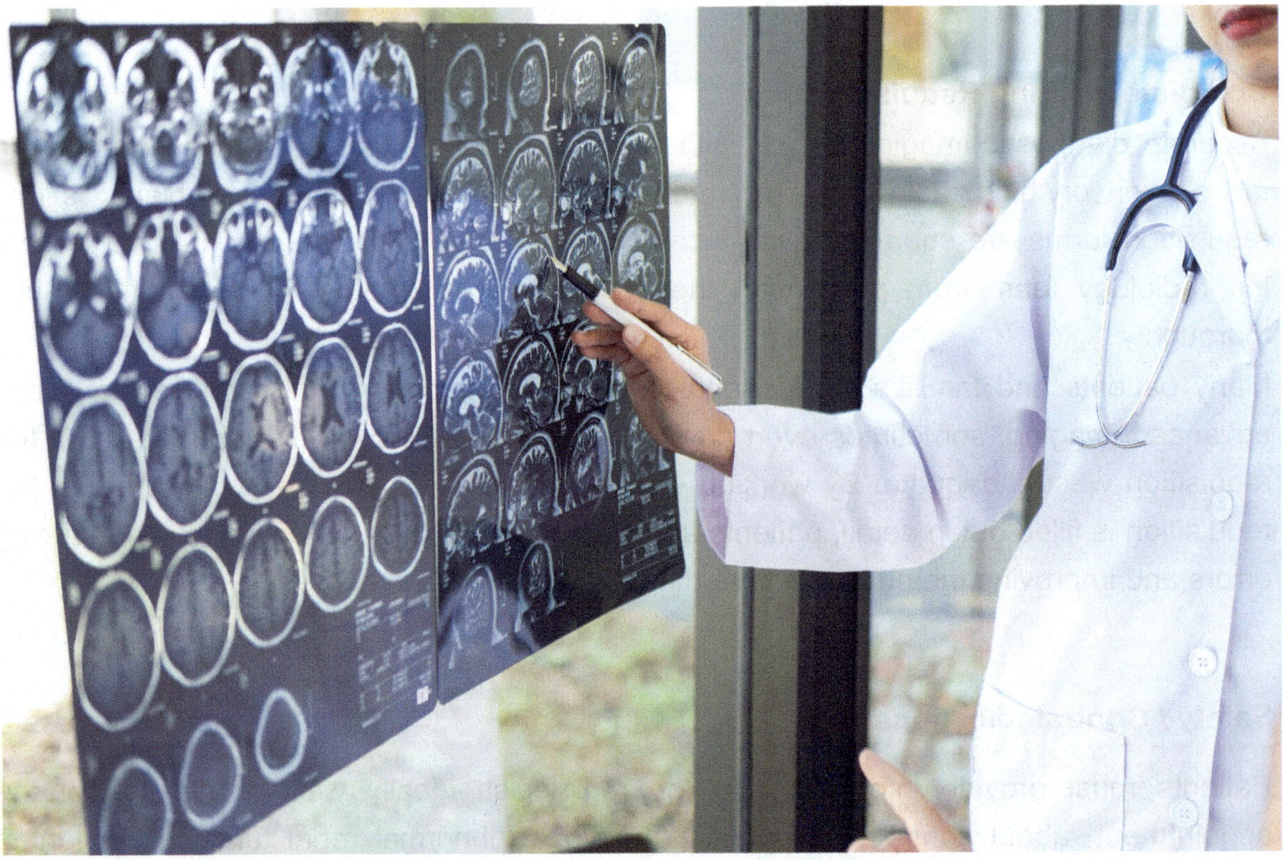

How Radiologists Look for Signs of CCI

Radiologists who specialize in disorders of the craniocervical junction look for specific indicators of abnormal movement, called radiology indicators of craniocervical instability (CCI). These are explained later in the section Overview of Radiology Indicators.

A radiologist experienced in CCI may see signs of instability on both supine scans (taken while lying down) and dynamic scans (taken while the neck is moving). In some patients, supine imaging appears normal, but dynamic MRI or CT scans reveal instability when the neck is placed in certain positions, such as flexion (bending forward), extension (bending back), rotation (turning side to side), or side-bending (tilting ear to shoulder).

CCI can involve abnormal movement of the skull and upper neck bones, including:

- Occiput–C1 (skull to first vertebra)
- C1–C2 (first and second vertebrae, also called atlantoaxial instability)
- Occiput–C2 (skull through second vertebra)
- Below C2 (subaxial instability)

Instability may occur in one or more directions:

- Vertical (up–down)
- Horizontal (front–back or side-to-side (lateral shift))
- Rotational (twisting movement)

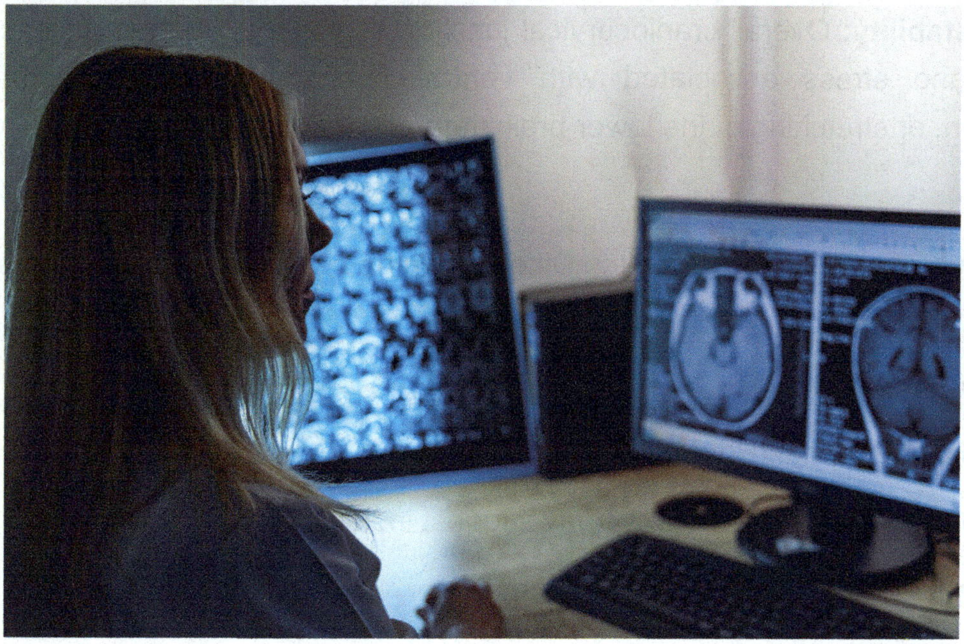

Overview of Radiology Indicators

The following radiology measurements are based on current peer-reviewed research. These measurements may be interpreted differently depending on the doctor's experience. For the most accurate and up-to-date information, always consult a specialist familiar with CCI, such as a CCI-knowledgeable radiologist or neurosurgeon.

Clivo-axial Angle (CXA)

The CXA measures the alignment of the clivus (a portion of the skull base) and the second vertebra (C2) of the upper cervical spine. Abnormalities in this angle may indicate misalignment or instability, which may stretch the brainstem and spinal cord and cause neurological symptoms. A few studies have found that a smaller CXA was associated with more severe neurological symptoms and higher disability scores.

Area of Instability: Overall craniocervical junction alignment. Used to assess brainstem deformity and stress associated with ventral brainstem *angulation*, and kinking, compression, or stretching of the lower brainstem and upper cervical spinal cord.

Neutral CXA Measurements: Note: Different authors may use slightly different cutoff values.

- Normal: 150° – 170°
- Mildly Abnormal (Borderline): 136° – 149°
- Abnormal: >170° or ≤ 135° (may suggest instability)
- Kyphotic CXA ≤ 124°

Dynamic CXA Measurements:

Some neurosurgeons use dynamic CXA measurements to detect instability not seen on neutral imaging. Research on dynamic MRI flexion (chin towards chest) and extension (chin upwards / head back) imaging is relatively new and small, and not widely understood at this time. Many more studies are needed, however, one small study indicated:

- Flexion CXA Normal Range: 134° - 163°
- Extension CXA Normal Range: 152° - 179°

When to Consult a Neurosurgeon: If the CXA is abnormal, a consultation with a neurosurgeon, especially if neurological symptoms are present is necessary. For a borderline measurement, it does not automatically mean surgery is necessary unless there are additional signs of progressive instability or clinical symptoms requiring intervention, yet it is crucial for patients to consult with a neurosurgeon for a full assessment.

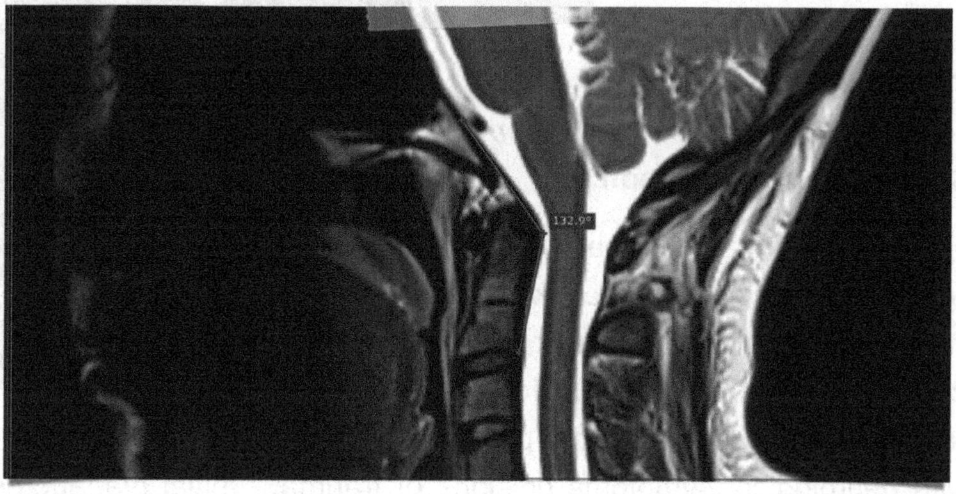

CXA

Powers Ratio

The Powers Ratio is a radiographic measurement used to assess instability at the junction between the skull and the first cervical vertebra (C1). It specifically helps detect anterior atlanto-occipital dislocation, a potentially serious condition requiring prompt evaluation.

Since 1979, the Powers Ratio has been widely used by radiologists, orthopaedic surgeons, and neurosurgeons to screen for atlanto-occipital dislocation and anterior horizontal instability.

However, it has limitations including it is *not* reliable for identifying posterior to dislocation and vertical distraction injuries (when spinal bones are forcefully pulled apart, typically due to high-energy trauma.)

Area of Instability: Anterior atlanto-occipital dislocation (AAOD)

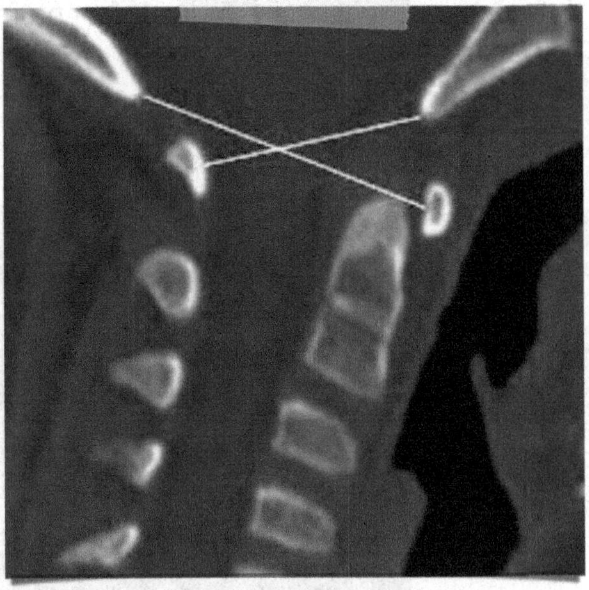

Neutral Reference Values:

- Normal:
  - ≤ 0.9
- Abnormal:
  - > 1.0

When to Consult a Neurosurgeon:

If the Powers Ratio is abnormal, it may indicate significant instability at the skull–C1 junction and should be treated as a potential emergency. Neurosurgical evaluation is strongly recommended, especially if the patient presents with neurological symptoms or signs of trauma. Initial management includes immediate cervical stabilization using a halo vest or hard cervical collar to prevent further injury.

Harris Measurements: BDI and BAI

Firmly established in the 1990s, the Harris measurements Basion-Dens Interval (BDI) and Basion-Axial Interval (BAI) are radiographic tools, often used together, to assess craniocervical junction stability, particularly at the skull to upper cervical spine region. These measurements help identify abnormal motion or displacement between the skull and the upper cervical spine.

Basion-Dens Interval (BDI)

Area of Instability: A key measurement to check stability between the skull and upper neck (craniocervical junction), specifically to evaluate how well the skull is aligned with the upper cervical spine, particularly with the second neck vertebra, known as C2. It helps detect conditions where the skull may be settling downward or separating from the spine, which could place pressure on the brainstem or spinal cord.

Neutral Reference Values:

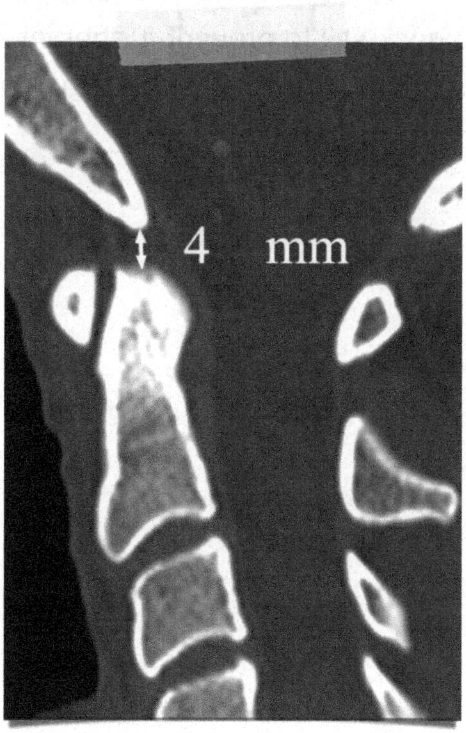

- Normal:

  < 12 mm on X-Rays (Less precise imaging modality)

  < 8.5 mm on CT

- Abnormal:

  > 12 mm on X-Rays (≥ 10 mm borderline abnormal)

  ≥ 8.5 mm on CT Scan

  ≥ 9 mm MRI (less precise compared to CT)

BDI Measurements on Dynamic Upright MRI Study:

A small 2023 Australian dynamic, upright MRI (uMRI) study stated the Basion-dens interval (BDI) did not exhibit a statistically significant difference when switching from neutral to flexion, suggesting that the reference values for BDI should not change much with the neck in neutral and flexion positions. The study demonstrated normal BDI ranges on uMRI as follows, however, such findings are not yet validated widely, and much more research is needed:

Neutral: 3 mm – 9 mm; mean (average) 5 mm

Flexion: 2.5 mm – 11 mm; mean 5 mm

Extension: 3 mm – 9.5 mm; mean 5.6 mm

Note: CT is preferred for accurate bony measurements. MRI is helpful for soft tissue (ligament) evaluation but is less reliable for bony measurements.

When to Consult a Neurosurgeon:

If the BDI is abnormal, patients should consider consulting with a neurosurgeon. Physicians may use a neck brace to keep the head and neck still to prevent further injury. In some cases, surgery may be needed to fuse the bones in the neck and head together to provide stability.

Dynamic Radiologic Measurements are not yet validated widely, and more research is needed.

Basion-Axial Interval (BAI)

Area of Instability: One of the key measurements used by doctors to assess the stability of the upper neck, especially where the base of the skull connects with the spine. Specifically, the BAI shows whether the skull is properly aligned with the second cervical vertebra (C2) such as, if the skull shifts too far forward (anterior) or backward (posterior) compared to C2, it may indicate instability, which can put pressure on the brainstem or upper spinal cord.

Neutral Reference Values:

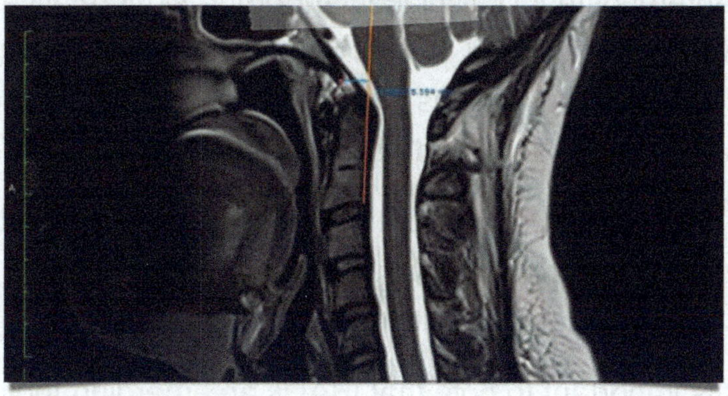

- Normal:

  < 12 mm (anterior)

  < 4 mm (posterior)

- Abnormal:

  ≥ 12 mm anterior displacement

  Posterior displacement ≥ 4 mm

BAI Measurements on Dynamic Upright MRI Study:

A small 2023 Australian dynamic, upright MRI (uMRI) study stated the Basion-axial interval (BAI) demonstrated normal BAI ranges on uMRI, however, such findings are not yet validated widely, and much more research is needed. Normal BAI ranges were as follows:

Neutral: 1 mm – 9.5 mm; mean 4.7 mm
Flexion: 0.5 mm – 11 mm; mean 5.5 mm
Extension: 0 mm – 8.5 mm; mean 3.2 mm

When to Consult a Neurosurgeon:

If the BAI is ≥ 12 mm or posterior displacement of ≥ 4 mm or more, patients should consider consulting with a neurosurgeon. Physicians may use a neck brace to keep the head and neck still to prevent further injury. In some cases, surgery may be needed to fuse the bones in the neck and head together to provide stability.

Emerging Dynamic Assessment using Translational BAI

The Basion-Dens Interval (BDI) is a well-established measurement, known as part of the Harris measurements, used by neurosurgeons and radiologists to assess vertical alignment between the base of the skull and the upper cervical spine. It plays an important role in identifying conditions like cranial settling and vertical instability.

Dynamic flexion-extension imaging allows measurement of how traditional indices like BDI and BAI vary with neck motion. Translational BAI (tBAI) assesses horizontal (anteroposterior) displacement of the skull relative to the spine, commonly by comparing BAI in flexion and extension. Translational BDI (tBDI) evaluates vertical displacement changes, but remains experimental and less validated. These dynamic measurements are investigational and not yet standard clinical practice.

These dynamic measurements help determine if the bones at the base of the skull and top of the neck move more than they should during motion, potentially indicating craniocervical instability (CCI).

It is important to note that tBAI is an emerging tool with some support from recent studies, suggesting that excessive motion (>2 mm) between positions may reflect instability. It is not yet standardized but is gaining recognition in surgical decision-making. tBDI is still experimental and not widely adopted or validated by clinical research.

Translational BAI is an emerging tool.

More research is needed on dynamic translational measurements.

Translational Basion-Axial Interval (tBAI)

Area of Instability: Translational Basion-Axial Interval (tBAI) measures changes in the BAI between flexion and extension positions, assessing horizontal (anteroposterior) instability. This dynamic assessment can reveal instability not evident on static neutral imaging. tBAI is still an emerging tool and not yet a standard part of diagnostic guidelines. More research is needed to confirm its accuracy and reliability in guiding treatment.

Reference Value Guidelines:

- Normal: ≤ 1 mm change between flexion and extension.
- Borderline abnormal: > 2 mm to ≤ 4 mm (Consider clinical correlation)
- Abnormal / possible instability: > 4 mm change, especially if symptomatic.

When to Consult a Neurosurgeon:

If translational BAI changes > 2 mm, particularly if > 4 mm and the patient presents with neurological symptoms (brainstem, cranial nerve, spinal cord, or autonomic) correlating with imaging, especially in cases involving connective tissue disorders, trauma, down syndrome with suspected instability.

For example, if a patient has the following dynamic BAI measurements: BAI in flexion (head down): 9 mm BAI in extension (head up): 5 mm tBAI = BAI in flexion – BAI in extension tBAI = 9 mm – 5 mm = 4 mm tBAI

Grabb-Oakes Line (GOL)

The Grabb-Oakes Line, first described by Grabb et al. in 1999, is a radiographic measurement used to assess ventral (underside) brainstem compression, particularly in patients with Chiari malformation. It determines the distance between the basion (base of the skull) and the C2 vertebra. Early dynamic studies have shown that GOL measurements remain stable across positions in neutral and flexion.

Area of Instability: CCI with brainstem compression

Neutral Reference Values:

- Normal: < 6 mm
- Borderline: 6 mm to 8 mm
- Abnormal: ≥ 9 mm; some use ≥ 8 mm

BDI Measurements on Dynamic Upright MRI Study:

Several small studies, including the 2023 Australian dynamic, upright MRI (uMRI) show minimal variation in GOL across neutral and flexion positions. The Australian study demonstrated normal GOL ranges on uMRI as follows, however, more research and validated dynamic standards are needed:

Neutral: 4.5 mm – 11 mm; mean (average) 7.2 mm
Flexion: 2.5 mm – 10.5 mm; mean 7.2 mm
Extension: 3 mm – 10.5 mm; mean 5.9 mm

When to Consult a Neurosurgeon:

If the neutral GOL measurement is greater than 8 mm, a neurosurgical evaluation is needed to explore potential treatment options.

Condylar–C1 Interval

The condylar-C1 interval measures the distance between each occipital condyle (the rounded bony knobs at the base of the skull) and the matching joint surface on C1 (the atlas). It helps detect instability where the skull may move abnormally on the top vertebra. It is an important finding after trauma, in connective-tissue disorders, or when joint degeneration occurs.

Area of Instability: Atlanto-occipital instability or injury

Reference Values (Measured on high-resolution CT i.e., < 1 mm slice thickness)

- **Normal:** ≤ 1.5 mm at each joint is generally considered normal.
- **Borderline:** approaching 1.5 mm or small asymmetry between sides should raise caution and prompt careful review.
- **Abnormal:** > 1.5 mm, or a condylar sum (left + right) > 3.0 mm, is strongly suggestive of abnormality and possible atlanto-occipital injury/instability.

Note: In addition to measuring the Condylar–C1 Interval, radiologists and specialists may also look for sliding (translational) movement between the skull and C1, uneven spacing (asymmetry) between left and right joints, or wear-and-tear changes (joint degeneration). On dynamic imaging (scans taken in flexion and extension), they can see if the joints gap or lose contact (facet gapping). They also check how well the skull and C1 surfaces still touch each other (facet apposition/overlap) as a reduced overlap may mean instability.

When to consult a neurosurgeon

If the condylar-C1 interval is >1.5 mm, or if the condylar sum >3.0 mm, or any abnormalities found in between the skull and C1, a neurosurgical consultation is recommended.

Atlanto-Dental Interval (ADI)

The atlanto-dental interval is the space between the first neck bone (C1) and the front of the second neck bone (C2) and if the space is too large, it may mean there's instability or a problem like ligament damage.

Area of Instability: Atlanto-axial joint (C1-C2)

Reference Values:

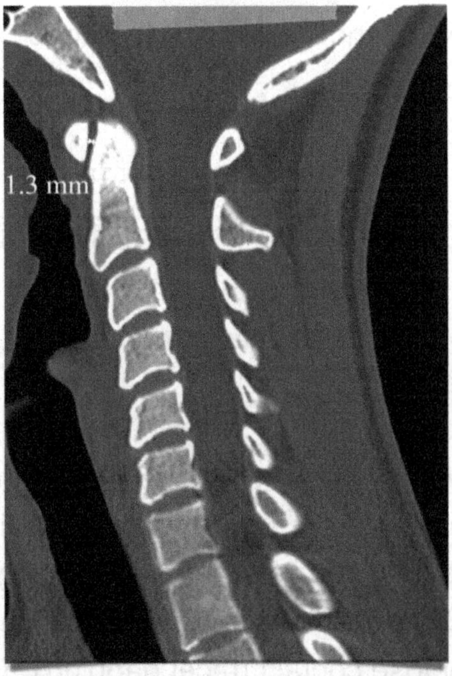

- Normal Values:
    - < 2 mm on CT scan
    - < 3 mm on radiograph
- Borderline Abnormal Values:
    - 2 mm – 4 mm may indicate potential instability, particularly if accompanied by risk factors such as trauma, connective tissue disease, or neurologic symptoms. Dynamic CT imaging is warranted.
- Abnormal Values:
    - ≥ 5 mm: Widely accepted as pathologic
    - ≥ 7 mm: Suggests rupture or incompetence of the transverse ligament. Indicates significant instability and potential risk for spinal cord compression

When to Consult a Neurosurgeon

If the ADI is > 2 mm, a neurosurgical consultation is recommended. Higher values (e.g., > 7 mm) may require urgent intervention to prevent further instability.

Sum of Lateral Mass Displacement (LMD)

Also known as Lateral Mass Overhang

Lateral Mass Displacement (LMD), also called lateral mass overhang, refers to the horizontal offset of the C1 (atlas) lateral masses beyond the margins of the C2 (axis) articular pillars. It is a classic radiographic indicator used to assess atlantoaxial instability, particularly rupture of the transverse ligament.

Static, open-mouth odontoid (anteroposterior) cervical X-ray in a neutral head position is the standard technique for applying the Rule of Spence.

Advanced imaging includes upright cone beam CT (uCBCT) or upright CT can provide more detailed views of the atlantoaxial relationship, especially under physiological load or movement. Open-mouth lateral side bending left and right, (With patient's ear to shoulder), can detect lateral mass displacement in dynamic positions.

Note: The Rule of Spence is based on the combined lateral overhang of both C1 lateral masses relative to C2 in static, neutral position. If the total overhang exceeds 6.9 mm, it suggests rupture of the transverse ligament. It was originally based on *cadaver studies,* and while still referenced today, its accuracy in living patients remains limited, highlighting the need for more clinical studies using live imaging.

Area of Instability: Atlanto-axial joint (C1–C2), focusing on the lateral masses

Reference Values:

- Normal: Less than 3 mm on one side
- Abnormal: A total overhang (left + right) > 6.9 mm suggests transverse ligament rupture.

When to Consult a Neurosurgeon:

If the Rule of Spence measurement exceeds 6.9 mm, dynamic MRI and CT studies and a neurosurgical evaluation are recommended.

Odontoid Lateral Mass Interval (OLMI)

The Odontoid-Lateral Mass Interval (OLMI) assesses the distance between the odontoid process (dens) of C2 and the lateral masses of the C1 vertebra. However, OLMI asymmetry can be a normal anatomical variation, especially in individuals with a side head tilt. Studies have shown that this asymmetry is more pronounced during head tilt than during head rotation, suggesting that positional factors influence the measurement. Isolated OLMI asymmetry, without associated clinical signs such as torticollis or cervical tenderness, may not require further investigation.

Area of Instability: Atlanto-axial joint (C1–C2)

Reference Values:

- Normal: Less than 5 mm
- Abnormal: Greater than 5 mm (right or left side)

Note: This abnormal value may appear in some medical sources but is not standardized across neurosurgical practice. OLMI is not a commonly used standalone diagnostic metric and further testing is necessary.

When to Consult a Neurosurgeon:

If the OLMI is greater than 5 mm, on the left or right side, it *may* indicate instability between the dens (C2) and lateral masses, and a further dynamic imaging studies are recommended.

Angles of Lateral Rotation (C1–C2)

The angles of right and left lateral rotation of the atlanto-axial joint (C1–C2) are used to evaluate rotational movement between the first and second cervical vertebrae, meaning, how far C1 can rotate relative to C2, and it is usually described as degrees of rotation per side. This measurement can help in diagnosing atlanto-axial instability, ligament injury, or abnormal stiffness. While valuable, it is important to note that reference cutoffs are **not universally standardized** and remain somewhat controversial.

Area of Instability: Atlanto-axial joint (C1–C2)

Reference Values (based on cadaveric and CT studies):

- **Normal:** ~31° per side
- **Borderline:** 35° - 40° per side
- **Pathological threshold (instability):** ≥ 40° per side (on CT axial views) (*Note: some references cite > 45° as the cut off value.)

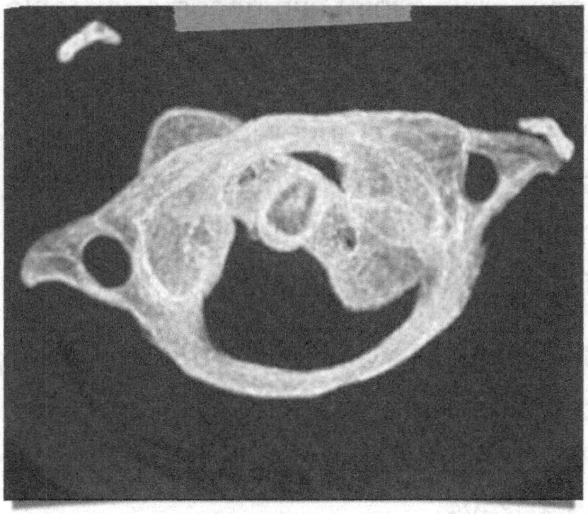

When to Consult a Neurosurgeon:

When rotational angles are abnormal, asymmetric, or associated with neurological symptoms, neurosurgical consultation is recommended.

Note: Exact numeric reference values vary between studies so the angles of lateral rotation measurement is highly controversial and not standardized. Reference Value alone is not diagnostic by itself and must be correlated with clinical and imaging context.

Understanding the Uniqueness of the Atlantoaxial Joint

The atlantoaxial joint is the connection between the first two bones in your neck, the atlas (C1) and the axis (C2). This joint is unlike any other in your spine. It acts like a swivel, allowing your head to turn side to side.

Almost half of all your head's rotation happens here. Because this joint needs to be so flexible, it also means it's inherently less stable than other parts of the spine. It depends heavily on strong ligaments, proper alignment of the small facet joints, and the shape of the bones to keep it in place.

Sometimes, due to physical trauma, loose ligaments, genetic conditions, arthritis, or wear and tear, this joint can become unstable. That means the bones may shift or slide in ways they shouldn't, either visibly or in subtle, hard-to-see ways.

When the small facet joints between C1 and C2 start to lose alignment, it can lead to facet dislocation or subluxation (bones slipping out of place), or a more hidden type of instability called Atlantoaxial Facet Subluxation or Central / Axial Atlantoaxial Instability (CAAD), where the joint looks normal on regular scans, but still moves abnormally.

Because the brainstem and spinal cord pass through this area, even small shifts can lead to symptoms like headaches, neck pain, dizziness, vision changes, or trouble thinking clearly. These issues can be missed if imaging is only done in a still (neutral) position or on X-Rays.

Doctors trained in this area may use dynamic imaging, like specialized 3D MDCT scans or CBCTs, taken while the head is in neutral, flexion, extension, lateral side bending, and rotation left and right, to see how the joint behaves and not just how it looks when resting.

Atlantoaxial Facet Subluxation / Dislocation

Atlantoaxial facet subluxation or dislocation often refers to a visible malalignment or dislocation of the C1–C2 facet joints on thin-sliced 3D CT in neutral and rotation CT to detect rotatory subluxation or fixation.

It may be a partial (subluxation) or complete dislocation, and can be due to traumatic, congenital or acquired (such as in rheumatoid arthritis, Grisel's syndrome, or connective tissue disorders).

Atlantoaxial facet subluxation or dislocation implies clear radiographic evidence based on advanced 3D high resolution CT/CBCT scans of malposition of the facets.

Atlantoaxial facet subluxation/dislocation is a clinically important, well-recognized entity in spine and neurosurgical fields, though its terminology and diagnostic criteria can vary somewhat across specialties.

Reference Values:

Normal: Facet joint displacement ≤ 2 mm, and/or rotational movement symmetry

Abnormal: > 2 mm indicates atlantoaxial subluxation; and/or rotational fixation or asymmetry suggesting joint locking or instability

When to Consult a Neurosurgeon

If imaging shows facet joint displacement greater than 2 mm and/or reveals rotational fixation or asymmetry of the atlantoaxial joints, with symptoms such as neck pain, limited neck movement, or neurological symptoms, a neurosurgical consultation with a CCI or atlantoaxial instability (AAI) specialist is recommended. Consultation is important to prevent further joint damage.

Atlantoaxial Rotary Instability

Atlantoaxial rotary instability (AARI) happens when the joint between the first cervical vertebra (C1, the atlas) and the second cervical vertebra (C2, the axis) becomes unstable during rotation of the head and neck. This joint is crucial for turning the head side to side. If too much of the joint surface "slides out of place" (contact loss), it may mean the joint is unstable.

Area of Instability: Atlantoaxial joint (facets)

Reference Values:

- Normal: < 80% contact loss
- Borderline: ≥80% contact loss
- Abnormal: ≥85% contact loss

When to Consult a Neurosurgeon:

You should seek neurosurgical consultation if imaging shows ≥ 80% facet contact loss at the C1–C2 joint.

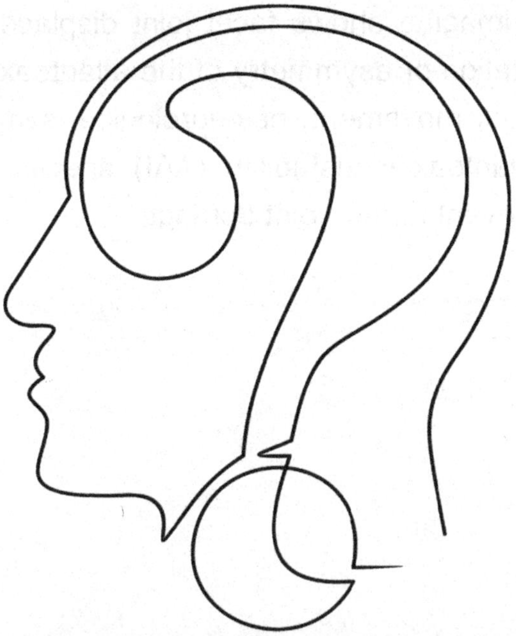

Dynamic Central or Axial Atlantoaxial Instability

This concept has been developed and widely used by Dr. Atul Goel, a globally recognized neurosurgeon and expert in atlantoaxial instability. His surgical techniques, based on diagnosing and stabilizing CAAD, have been adopted by neurosurgeons in various countries. However, it's important to note that the CAAD classification remains an emerging concept and is not yet widely adopted in some neurosurgical literature or included in international diagnostic standards.

Central or Axial Atlantoaxial Instability (CAAD) refers to instability at the C1–C2 (atlantoaxial) joint, specifically involving abnormal alignment or subtle slipping (subluxation) of the facet joints between the atlas (C1) and axis (C2).

This form of instability may not always be visible on standard imaging and is sometimes called **"Occult Atlantoaxial Instability".**

CAAD is typically assessed using high resolution dynamic CT imaging in neutral, flexion, extension and rotation views, to allow clinicians to evaluate whether the C1 and C2 facet joints are properly aligned in different positions. A misalignment greater than 3 mm is generally considered abnormal.

Dynamic imaging may reveal subtle facet joint movement that static scans miss, supporting the value of advanced dynamic imaging in detecting "hidden" instability on basic imaging.

Area of Instability: Atlantoaxial facet joints (C1–C2)

Reference Values:

Normal: Facets are properly aligned < 3mm

Abnormal: Facet joint misalignment ≥ 3 mm

When to Consult a Neurosurgeon:

If there is facet joint misalignment or suspected occult instability, especially when symptoms such as neck pain, headaches, or neurological issues are present, consulting a neurosurgeon experienced in atlanto-axial instability disorders is recommended.

Other Potential Radiology Imaging Indicators

Imaging plays a key role in identifying abnormalities in the upper neck, especially at the craniocervical junction. This joint is highly mobile and especially vulnerable to injury or degeneration. Even subtle misalignments or wear-and-tear in this area can be linked to neck pain, dizziness, headaches, tinnitus (ringing in the ears), and nerve-related symptoms like arm pain or facial pressure.

Some of the imaging signs of degeneration or injury may include:

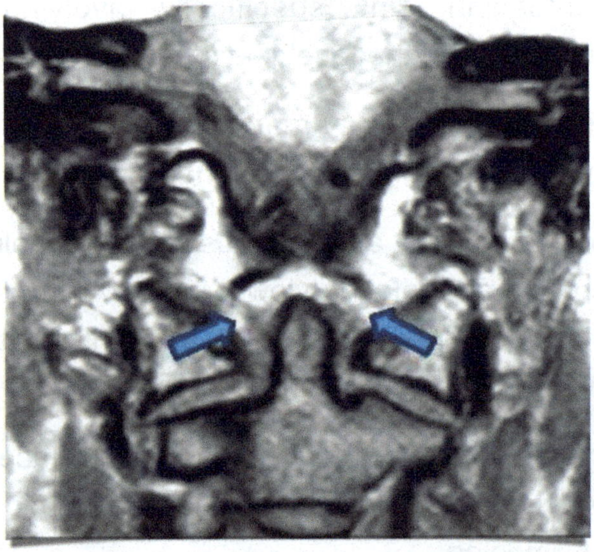

- Joint space narrowing (loss of normal spacing between joints)
- Subchondral sclerosis (hardening of bone under the joint surface)
- Osteophyte formation (bone spurs or overgrowths)
- Facet cysts, sometimes calcified
- Capsular thickening (inflammation or fibrosis of the joint lining)
- Ligament ossification (the ligament becomes abnormally hard)
- Ligament and membrane injury (3T MRI assessment of craniocervical junction ligaments) such as the alar, transverse and anterior atlanto-occipital membrane
- Spinal Canal Stenosis (via canal dimensions or signs of crowding of the spinal cord)
- Interspinous Distance, malalignment etc.
- Foraminal Stenosis or grading

Because some of these findings are subtle, it's important for physicians and radiologists whenever possible to use high-resolution 3D imaging, such as dynamic CT scans or cone-beam CT (CBCT) and 1.5T or 3T MRI of the craniocervical junction studies. Interpreting these scans carefully helps doctors detect small yet meaningful signs of instability or joint dysfunction that may explain a patient's symptoms and lead to more accurate diagnosis and treatment.

Cervical Spondylotic Myelopathy

Patients with a condition called cervical spondylotic myelopathy with or without instability, which is when age-related wear, disc damage, or instability in the neck causes pressure on the spinal cord, often have more severe wear-and-tear in their neck joints.

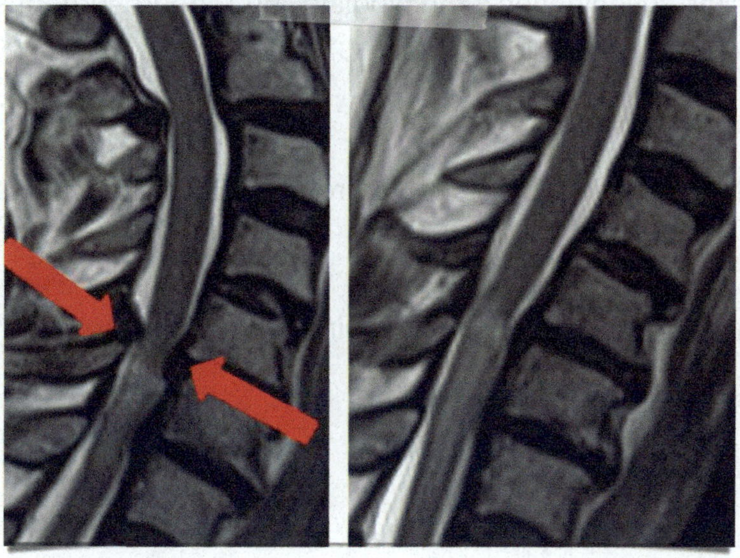

Loss of Cervical Lordosis

Loss of cervical lordosis, often called "straight neck," can disrupt normal spinal alignment and increase stress on cervical facet joints. A systematic review and meta-analysis of cervical spine alignment found the average cervical lordosis angle to be approximately 16.9 degrees. Moderate loss of cervical lordosis (10°–20°) may reduce CSF and vertebral artery flow, while severe loss (<10°) or reversal (kyphosis) carries a higher risk of clinically significant flow disruption. More studies are needed.

Maintaining this normal curvature is essential for spinal health, as deviations from it can lead to various spinal disorders, including increased strain on the facet joints and progressive development of degenerative conditions.

Chamberlain's Line (Dens over Chamberlain)

Basilar invagination (BI) is a structural abnormality where the upper part of the cervical spine (especially the odontoid process or dens) moves upward into the base of the skull. This displacement may compress the brainstem, upper spinal cord, or surrounding neurovascular structures, leading to neurological symptoms.

To assess for basilar invagination, radiologists and neurosurgeons rely on several craniometric lines on imaging studies (usually CT or MRI):

1. Chamberlain's Line

Normal: The tip of the odontoid (dens) should project < 3 mm above this line.

Abnormal:

> >3 mm: Suggests possible basilar invagination (borderline)
>
> >5 mm: Considered clearly abnormal

2. McGregor's Line

Normal: The dens should not project more than:

> 4.5 mm in males
>
> 10 mm in females

3. McRae's Line

Normal: The tip of the dens should be located below this line.

Abnormal: If the dens projects above McRae's line, it indicates basilar invagination.

When to Consult a Neurosurgeon:

If the measurement is abnormal, a neurosurgical evaluation is recommended.

Chiari Malformation

Tonsillar Herniation / Descent

Tonsillar descent or tonsillar herniation means that part of the lower brain (called the cerebellar tonsils) is hanging down lower than it should and below the opening at the bottom of the skull (called the foramen magnum). This can sometimes press on nearby nerves or the spinal cord.

The measurement of the downward displacement of the cerebellar tonsils below the foramen magnum is commonly referred to as tonsillar descent or tonsillar herniation. This assessment is crucial in diagnosing *Chiari Malformation*. It's important to note that the degree of tonsillar descent alone may not correlate directly with symptom severity, and clinical correlation is necessary.

It's also important to note that there is ongoing controversy in the diagnosis of Chiari malformation due to lack of consensus on measurement thresholds, the clinical relevance of tonsillar descent, and the role of CSF flow studies, leading to variability in both diagnosis and treatment decisions.

Why Chiari Isn't Just About Measurements

A 2019 study titled *Chiari I Malformation: Opinions on Diagnostic Trends and Controversies* surveyed 63 international experts. The study found that most experts no longer rely on the traditional "5-mm rule," which defines Chiari malformation based solely on a 5 mm or more drop of the cerebellar tonsils. Instead, 88.5% agreed that this measurement alone is not enough for diagnosis.

The experts emphasized that a patient's symptoms and other imaging results are just as important, sometimes more so than the tonsil measurement. This marks a shift toward a more personalized approach to diagnosis and treatment, focusing on how the condition affects each person individually. Patients should work closely with knowledgeable specialists to fully evaluate their symptoms and imaging findings for the best care plan.

"Complex Chiari" malformation is a term specialists use to describe chiari's tonsillar descent with the added involvement of associated bony, ligamentous, or neural abnormalities that can increase the risk of neurological compromise.

International Guidelines on Chiari Malformation 2023

The Congress of Neurological Surgeons (CNS), an international organization based in the USA, released updated guidelines for the management of Chiari Malformation Type I (CM-I) in 2023.

Key Points from the CNS 2023 Guideline on Chiari Malformation:

Tonsillar Descent Measurement:

- Tonsillar descent (downward displacement of the cerebellar tonsils) remains an essential diagnostic criterion for CM-I, with the threshold for abnormal descent still set at 5 mm or more below the foramen magnum.
- However, the guideline encourages clinicians to assess symptoms along with tonsillar descent, noting that some patients with descent between 3 and 5 mm might also exhibit clinical signs of CM, particularly when associated with syringomyelia (a fluid-filled cyst within the spinal cord) or abnormal CSF flow.
- Advanced imaging, including MRI and Cine MRI (i.e., a special type of MRI that shows how fluid flows in the brain and spine, almost like a video and in this context, it helps doctors see if the cerebrospinal fluid (CSF) is flowing properly around the brain and spinal cord, which is important when there is tonsillar descent or a syrinx (a fluid-filled cavity in the spinal cord).
- MRI and Cine MRI plays a critical role in assessing not only tonsillar descent but also CSF flow and any associated syringomyelia. These imaging findings help determine the necessity and timing of surgical intervention.

Is Atlantoaxial Instability The Cause Chiari Malformation?

Dr. Atul Goel, a renowned neurosurgeon specializing in craniovertebral junction disorders, who began his career in the field of neurosurgery in the 1980s, has proposed that atlantoaxial instability (AAI) is a primary cause of Chiari malformation (CM), and that stabilizing the atlantoaxial joint can effectively treat CM. His studies suggest that this approach can lead to significant improvements in symptoms and even resolution of associated conditions like syringomyelia.

In a 2015 study published in the Journal of Neurosurgery: Spine, Dr. Goel treated 65 patients with CM by performing atlantoaxial fixation. The results indicated that this

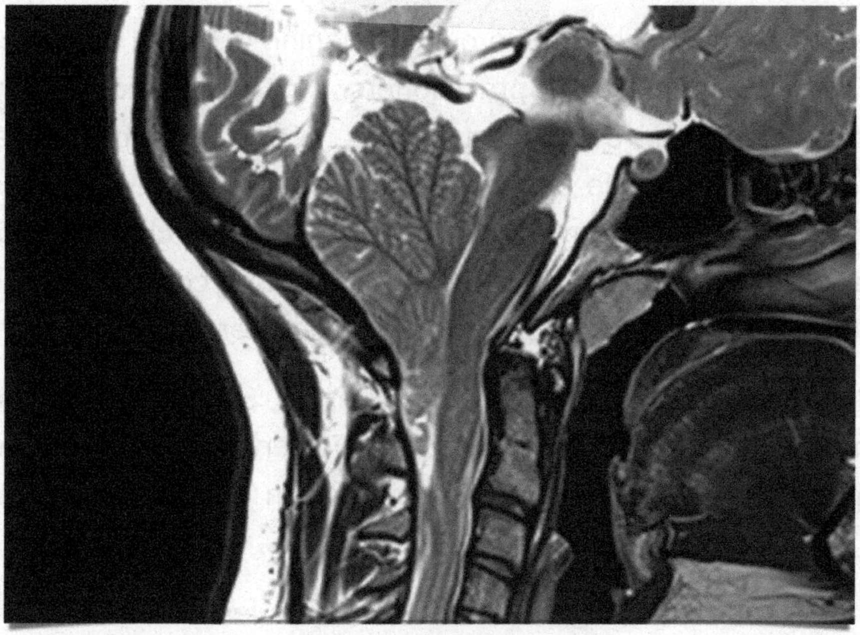

Chiari Malformation

surgical intervention could address the underlying instability, leading to symptomatic relief in many cases.

Further research by Dr. Goel, published in 2020 in the Journal of Craniovertebral Junction and Spine, examined 25 patients who had undergone foramen magnum decompression without success. These patients were subsequently treated with atlantoaxial fixation, resulting in improved neurological function and a reduction in syrinx size in several cases.

Dr. Goel's findings challenge traditional views that CM is primarily due to posterior fossa (small space at the back of the skull, near the base of the brain) abnormalities. Instead, he emphasizes the role of atlantoaxial instability and advocates for stabilization procedures as a treatment strategy.

While these studies present compelling evidence supporting atlantoaxial fixation in treating CM, the approach remains controversial and is not widely adopted. Further research and clinical trials are needed to validate these findings and determine the best treatment protocols for patients with CM.

CCI Comorbidities to Rule Out on Imaging

The following list of *comorbidities to rule out on imaging is based on clinical observation and emerging patterns reported by practitioners. Not all of these comorbidities are universally recognized in peer-reviewed guidelines. Other non-imaging related medical conditions to rule out may include connective tissue disorders, Lyme disease and other chronic infections, rheumatoid arthritis, ankylosing spondylitis, chronic inflammation, and mast cell activation syndrome, to name a few. Some CCI comorbidities to rule out on imaging, some of which will be briefly outlined in this chapter, include:

- Eagle Jugular Syndrome (similar medical terms Styloidogenic Jugular Venous Compression Syndrome (SJVCS) or Styloidogenic-cervical spondylotic internal jugular venous compression, or Atlanto-Styloid Compression Syndrome, or Vascular Eagles Syndrome)
- Cervical spinal stenosis (A sagittal canal diameter less than 10 mm is generally considered indicative of cervical spinal stenosis and increased risk of spinal cord compression; and cervical spondylosis (degeneration of the bones, discs, and joints)
- Loss of cervical lordosis (natural curvature)
- Signs of increased intracranial pressure / hypertension, and Hydrocephalus
- Structural brain changes and signs of neurological disease such as stroke, vascular dementia, Alzheimer's disease, Multiple Sclerosis, Cerebral Venous Sinus Thrombosis and Traumatic Brain Injury
- Compressed or stenosis of blood vessels
- Signs of disrupted CSF flow and blood circulation
- Ossification (hardening) of ligaments, and ligament or membrane tears
- Brainstem, and cranial nerve compression
- Cranial settling, and Basilar invagination
- Scoliosis, Platybasia, and Kyphosis
- Tethered Cord syndrome located in the lumbosacral (lower back) spine

Eagle Jugular Syndrome

Eagle Syndrome occurs when bone or ligament at the base of the skull or cervical spine press on nearby nerves and/or major blood vessels. The main structures involved in the compression of nerves and / or major blood vessels (such as the internal jugular vein or carotid artery), are the styloid process, the stylohyoid ligament, and the C1 (atlas) transverse process.

How compression can happen:

- The styloid process (a pointy bone from the base of the skull to beneath the ear) can be too long or thick, or its orientation can angle inwards, causing compression.
- The stylohyoid ligament can harden (ossify) into bone (a ligament located in the neck) and cause compression of nerves or blood vessels.
- The C1 transverse process (a part of the first vertebra) can impinge nerves or major blood vessels because of an abnormal shape or bone growth.
- In some cases other abnormalities such as surgical scarring, can contribute to compression.

Nearby, there are important cranial nerves (trigeminal, facial, glossopharyngeal, vagus), blood vessels (internal jugular vein, carotid artery), the sternocleidomastoid (SCM) muscle, and the pharynx, so symptoms can be varied.

Reported contributors include congenital factors, age-related calcification, trauma/ whiplash, repetitive mechanical stress, prior surgery (e.g., tonsillectomy), and pharyngeal infections linked to rheumatic styloiditis (inflammation leading to ossification). Genetic/ metabolic factors may play a role. Not everyone with an elongated styloid or ossified ligament has symptoms.

Most styloids are 1–3 cm; elongated is > 3 cm (or > 2.5 cm in women). Only a small percentage with elongation develop symptoms.

Eagle Syndrome Variants

1) Classic (Nerve-related) Eagle Syndrome

Irritation or compression of nearby cranial nerves.

- Symptoms: throat pain, ear pain (otalgia), neck/jaw/facial pain, trouble swallowing (dysphagia), globus (feeling something stuck), voice changes.
- Often worse with swallowing, chewing, or turning the head.

2) Vascular (Blood-vessel-related) Eagle Syndrome

Compression of veins or arteries.

Venous (IJV) compression, also called Venous Eagle / Styloidogenic Jugular Venous Compression Syndrome (SJVCS) / Eagle Jugular syndrome.

- Symptoms: pulsatile tinnitus, headaches, brain fog, visual disturbances, profound fatigue (often worse upright or with activity), dizziness/vertigo, sleep problems, ear/eye pressure, anxiety, depression, irritability, nausea, vomiting, transient vision loss, neck pain or tightness (often SCM).
- May present with intracranial hypertension (head pressure).
- Symptoms often worse with neck/head movements, and when lying down.

Arterial (carotid/vertebral) compression

- Symptoms: dizziness, transient weakness or numbness on one side, TIA-like episodes, and rarely stroke.

The elongated / misoriented styloid or ossified ligament impinges on C1 (or C1 itself is abnormally shaped or bony overgrowth), which can worsen venous/arterial or nerve compression.

Anterior subluxation of C1 (forward shift) can narrow the space for the internal jugular vein (J3 segment), especially with ligamentous laxity or loss of cervical lordosis (loss of normal neck curvature); and a surgically fused C1–C2 segment can impinge the IJV (bony overgrowth or hardware placement near the vein).

Eagle Jugular Syndrome (EJS) Radiology Assessment

A subtype of Eagle syndrome where an elongated or medially-angled styloid process (a thin bone that projects down from the skull base) presses against the internal jugular vein (IJV), often between the styloid and the transverse process or of C1. This can reduce blood flow from the brain to the heart, leading to head pressure symptoms, headaches, cognitive dysfunction, tinnitus, dizziness, visual disturbances, involuntary motor episodes or dysautonomia-like symptoms. EJS as gained increasing attention in medical literature over the past decade and is still considered a rare condition. More research on is needed.

Area of Abnormality: IJV at the site where the styloid and C1 come together

Best evaluated with high-resolution (< 1mm slice thickness) dual-phase (arterial and venous phases) 3D CT angiogram of neck vessels in neutral, and if possible, head rotated left and right positions.

Reference Values:

- **Styloid Length**
  - Normal: usually less than ~25–30 mm
  - Borderline: 25 mm - 30 mm (moderately long)
  - Abnormal: >30 mm (elongated styloid)
- **3-D Styloid Orientation**

Styloid orientation / angulation is still under research, however, researchers look not just at the length of the styloid bone but also how it is angled / oriented. If the styloid points more medially or downward toward the C1 vertebra, it can press on the internal jugular vein and reduce blood flow from the brain, even if the bone is only moderately long. In fact, studies of Eagle Jugular Syndrome emphasize that the medial angulation (toward the midline) and inferior/vertical orientation of the styloid are more important than length alone.

  - Normal orientation: Angles >75° tend to point laterally and are less likely to compress the vein.

- Abnormal orientation:
    - The styloid bone may point medially enough to approach or touch C1, creating a 'sandwich' effect on the internal jugular vein; this close positioning is called C1–Styloid juxtaposition.
    - Some morphometric studies describe angles < 65°–70° from midline as relatively more medially directed

- **Styloid–C1 distance:**
    - Normal: no close contact; measured shortest distance between styloid tip and C1 transverse process/lateral mass.
    - Borderline: 5 mm - 7.5 mm (warrants further clinical evaluation)
    - Abnormal / suspicious: < 5 mm between styloid tip and C1 has been reported as frequently associated with IJV compression.

- **Jugular vein narrowing:**
    - Clinically significant: reduction > 50% at the narrowest point compression is often considered (hemodynamically) relevant.

When to consult a Neurosurgeon or ENT specializing in Vascular Eagle (Jugular) Syndrome

Consult neurosurgery or a otolaryngology team experienced with C1-styloid related vascular compression if imaging shows a styloid–C1 distance ≤ 7.5 mm, medial angulation toward C1, or > 50% narrowing of the internal jugular vein, even if symptoms are mild.

Eagle Jugular Syndrome, Intracranial Pressure and Anxiety, Panic Attacks and Depression

Eagle syndrome (ES) can be caused by an abnormally long or misshapen styloid process or a calcified stylohyoid ligament, which can compress nearby structures such as blood vessels or nerves. This compression can cause symptoms like throat pain, a foreign body sensation in the throat, pain in the neck or jaw, vertigo, and even toothache.

In some cases, Eagle Jugular syndrome (EJS) can also compress the internal jugular veins, which may lead to increased venous congestion or intracranial pressure, resulting in symptoms such as headaches, visual disturbances, and psychiatric symptoms such as anxiety, panic attacks, and depression.

The vascular and psychological symptom connections are plausible but still somewhat emerging in research, however, some studies show that a significant number of EJS patients report psychological distress, and many experience relief of both physical and mental symptoms following surgical removal of the elongated styloid process.

Since ES and CCI can share overlapping symptoms, it is important to obtain imaging to assess for both conditions. Consultation with a neurosurgeon specializing in CCI, and an ENT specializing in ES is needed to ensure accurate diagnosis and appropriate treatment planning.

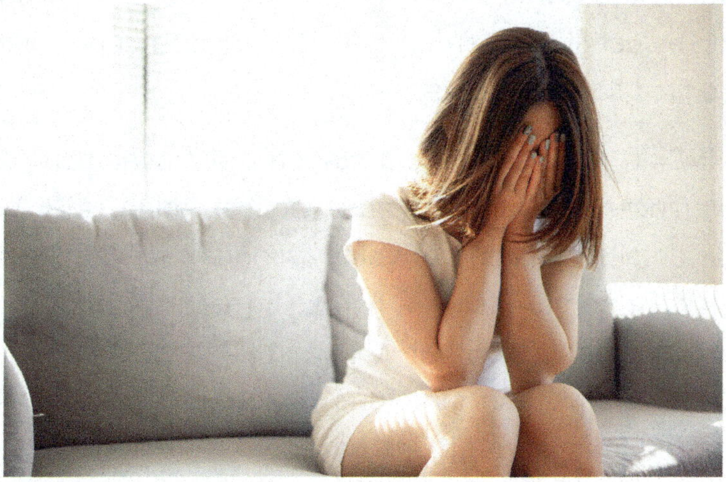

Note: Cases involving mental health symptoms, intracranial pressure, and psychological distress are reported but are derived from small observational case series, not large-scale trials. These findings are suggestive but not yet proven in broad populations. More research is needed.

Impact of CCJ Dysfunction on Brain Health

Blood and CSF Flow

CCI may, but not in all cases, affect blood flow and cerebrospinal fluid (CSF) dynamics in the neck and brain, potentially contributing to conditions involving venous congestion and increased intracranial pressure (ICP). However, these radiographic imaging findings are sometimes overlooked or considered incidental by general radiologists. CCI can compress blood vessels in the neck. In certain cases, it is important to carefully evaluate both vascular conditions in the head and neck, and CCI before proceeding with treatment.

Importantly, neck conditions such as spinal stenosis (narrowing of the spinal canal spaces that compress nerves or the spinal cord), cervical spondylosis (degenerative changes in the cervical spine) and loss of cervical lordosis (abnormal curvature in the neck) can directly disrupt CSF flow and blood circulation between the brain and spinal canal. These disruptions can exacerbate symptoms by altering normal CSF and blood dynamics.

An Analogy of CSF and Blood Flow

Imagine the brain is like a garden, and CSF and blood are the water it needs to stay healthy. If the hose (representing the CCJ) gets pinched or bent, the water may not flow properly. Some parts of the garden may flood (from pressure buildup), while others dry out (from lack of flow). Just like a garden gets damaged by poor watering, the brain can suffer from disrupted fluid flow over time.

Phase-Contrast MRI/Cine MRI is the gold standard for evaluating CSF and blood flow dynamics at the craniocervical junction and cervical spine. MR Venography and MR Angiography provide detailed imaging of veins (venous) and arteries (arterial) blood flow in the brain and neck. In some cases, CT imaging is also used to better assess bone structures or vascular anatomy. Together, MRI and CT techniques offer a comprehensive evaluation of CSF, blood flow, and structural abnormalities. However, physicians often have their own preferred imaging methods based on their specialty, experience, and the specific clinical situation, choosing the techniques that best suit each patient's needs.

Patients with imaging findings associated with blood and CSF flow abnormalities should consult specialists. Assessment for CSF or blood flow disruption is not routine, which is why cine-MRI, MRV, and MRA are often requested by specialists.

Radiologic signs to consider include:

- Bilateral Transverse Sinus Stenosis (TSSS): Narrowing of the transverse venous sinuses
- Sigmoid Sinus Dehiscence: Thinning or absence of bone over the sigmoid sinus
- Optic Nerve Tortuosity: Abnormal twisting or bending of the optic nerves
- Optic Disc Protrusion: Bulging of the optic disc into the eye socket

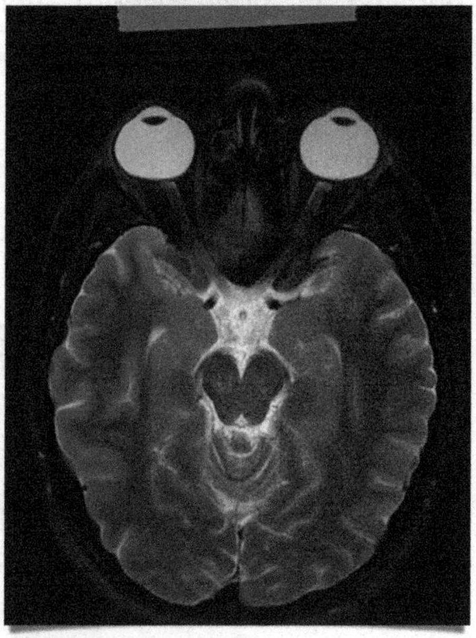

- Optic Canal Changes: Enlargement or erosion of the optic canal over time in patients with chronic untreated IIH
- Tortuosity of Blood Vessels: Twisted or curved blood vessels.
- Posterior Scleral Flattening: Flattening of the posterior portion of the eyeball
- Perioptic Subarachnoid Space (SAS) Dilatation: Enlargement of the space surrounding the optic nerve
- Empty Sella Syndrome: Flattening or partial collapse of the pituitary gland
- Meningocele: Protrusions of the meninges through defects in the skull or spine, related to pressure changes
- Spontaneous Cerebrospinal Fluid (CSF) Leaks: CSF leaks from the spinal canal that may contribute to IIH symptoms. Note: Not all spontaneous CSF leaks occur due to CCI or venous congestion, and not all patients with CCI develop leaks.
- Other structural brain changes

Structural Brain Changes

Abnormalities at the craniocervical junction can disrupt the normal flow of CSF and blood into and out of the brain. When this flow is blocked or slowed, it can cause increased intracranial pressure or reduce the delivery of oxygen and nutrients to brain tissue, as well as impair the removal of waste products.

Over time, these changes may lead to structural brain alterations such as atrophy (shrinking of brain tissue), ventricular enlargement (fluid-filled spaces in the brain expanding), white matter lesions, and depending on severity, duration, and other comorbid factors, may damage regions involved in memory, coordination, and balance. These structural changes may contribute to cognitive decline and neurological symptoms.

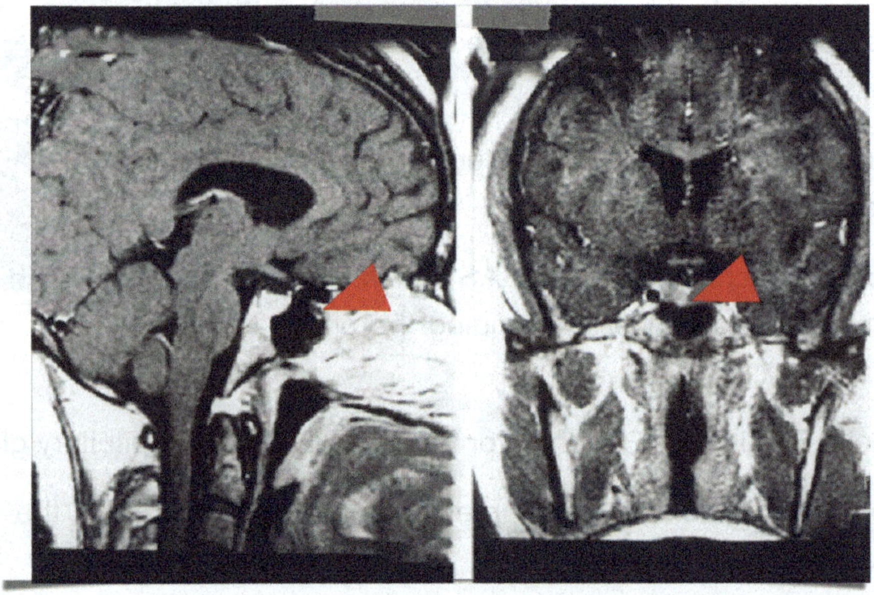

Empty Sella Syndrome on MRI Image

3 Tesla Magnetic Resonance Imaging (MRI) is the gold standard for detecting and monitoring these structural brain changes because it provides detailed images of brain tissue, ventricles, and white matter integrity.

It's important for the ordering physician to prepare an appropriate imaging requisition, for the radiology technician to use the right equipment and complete the correct imaging sequences, and the radiologist to be knowledgable, and complete a thorough and accurate report.

Study: How Increased Intracranial Pressure Can Affect Thinking and Memory

Increased ICP, such as in idiopathic intracranial hypertension (IIH), can affect how the brain functions and lead to cognitive problems. A clinical study found that patients with IIH performed worse than healthy individuals in several areas of cognitive function, especially reaction time and processing speed.

Even after treatment improved their ICP levels and reduced headaches, many patients still showed signs of cognitive difficulties three months later. This suggests that high ICP may have a lasting impact on brain function, which can interfere with daily tasks, memory, and overall mental clarity.

Analogy: Your Brain is Like a Busy City

Think of the brain like a busy city. The streets are like blood vessels, and cars carry oxygen and food to help the brain work. Thoughts and memories are like important packages being delivered around the city.

Now imagine a big rainstorm floods the city. Water fills the streets, and cars can't move easily. Traffic gets stuck, and the packages don't get where they need to go.

This is what happens when pressure inside the head gets too high. The brain can't work the way it should. Blood flow slows down, and brain cells don't get enough oxygen. This can make it hard to think clearly, remember things, or focus—just like a city that's flooded and stuck in traffic.

Brainstem Compression

Medical name: *Cervical Medullary Syndrome / Cervicomedullary Compression.*

When there are abnormalities in the craniocervical junction, such as misalignment, narrowing, or instability, they may lead to compression of the lowest part of the brainstem, particularly the *medulla oblongata*. This condition is often referred to as Cervical Medullary Syndrome, Cervicomedullary Compression, or simply Craniocervical Junction Compression.

The brainstem controls essential functions like breathing, heart rate, swallowing, and balance. Compression in this area can cause symptoms such as dizziness, difficulty swallowing, numbness, weakness, poor coordination, or breathing problems.

Dynamic MRI Cervical Spine and Craniocervical Junction in neutral, flexion and extension positions is an excellent imaging technique for assessing brainstem compression because it allows doctors to see how the craniocervical junction moves while upright and during different head positions, helping to identify instability or pressure on the brainstem that might not be visible on standard static scans.

Autonomic Dysfunction

Medical Name: *Dysautonomia.*

The brainstem and upper cervical spinal cord, located near the craniocervical junction, play a central role in controlling the autonomic nervous system which regulates involuntary functions like heart rate, blood pressure, digestion, and temperature control.

When abnormalities at the CCJ cause compression or instability, they can interfere with brainstem signaling and cranial nerve function such as the vagus nerve (which helps regulate heart rate, digestion, and other autonomic processes). This disruption may contribute to dysautonomia, with symptoms such as dizziness, fainting, rapid or slow heart rate (tachycardia or bradycardia), POTS (Postural Orthostatic Tachycardia Syndrome), poor temperature regulation, or gastrointestinal issues.

However, it's important to recognize that similar symptoms can also result from other conditions such as autoimmune disease, small fiber neuropathy, metabolic disorders, or primary dysautonomia. These differential diagnoses should be carefully considered and ruled out.

Spinal Cord Compression

Medical Name: *Myelopathy.*

The spinal cord passes through the craniocervical junction (CCJ) and serves as a vital communication pathway between the brain and the rest of the body. When abnormalities in the CCJ cause narrowing or misalignment, *the spinal cord may become compressed*, leading to a condition known as myelopathy and can easily been seen on imaging.

This may cause symptoms such as tingling, weakness, poor coordination, or difficulty walking. If left untreated, prolonged pressure can result in permanent spinal cord damage. It is typically at this stage of ongoing compression and neurological decline that all neurosurgeons will consider surgical intervention, such as spinal fusion, to prevent further injury.

Standard Magnetic Resonance Imaging (MRI) is considered the gold standard for diagnosing spinal cord compression and assessing the extent of myelopathy because it provides detailed images of soft tissues, including the spinal cord and surrounding structures, but dynamic MRI is an emerging adjunct for detecting *positional* cervical cord compression in cases of suspected instability.

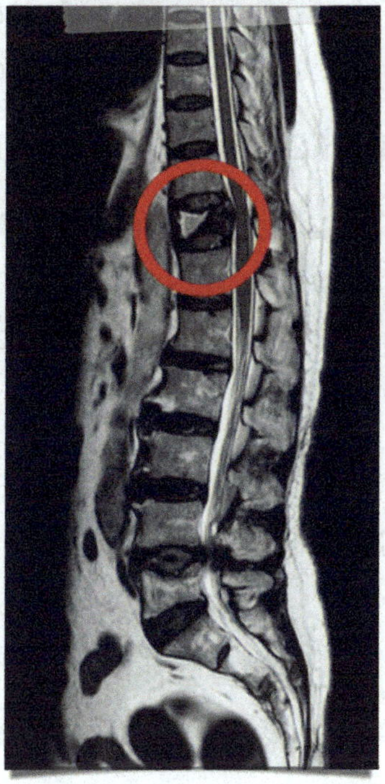

Spinal Cord Compression on MRI

Cranial Nerve Compression

Conditions like craniocervical instability, os odontoideum, basilar invagination, and Klippel-Feil syndrome can cause misalignment of the upper neck bones, putting pressure on cranial nerves that control speaking, swallowing, and facial movement. Other causes include joint degeneration, inflammation, cysts, or abnormal tissue growth.

Symptoms of nerve compression may include difficulty speaking or swallowing, facial pain, hoarseness, and weakness or poor coordination. Advanced MRI scans help detect nerve compression and identify causes. This aids neurosurgeons in deciding if surgery or other treatments are needed to relieve pressure and prevent further damage.

Brief Overview of the Cranial Nerves and Possible Symptoms

The 24 cranial nerves (CN), 12 on the left side and 12 on the right side, originating from the brain and brainstem, are responsible for essential motor and sensory functions in the head, neck, and body. Compression or irritation of these nerves can result in a wide range of symptoms, depending on which nerve is involved.

Common cranial nerve symptoms and possible implications include:

- **CN I: Olfactory:** The sense of smell nerve. Loss or alteration of smell (anosmia), which may affect taste perception.
- **CN II: Optic:** The vision nerve. Blurred vision, visual field loss, or double vision. It is actually part of the brain itself that carries visual information from the eyes to the brain. Doctors sometimes call it a tract of the central nervous system because it behaves more like a brain pathway than a typical peripheral nerve.
- **CN III: Oculomotor:** The eye movement nerve. Double vision, drooping eyelid (ptosis), pupil changes, or difficulty focusing.
- **CN IV: Trochlear:** Eye pulley movement nerve. Vertical double vision, trouble moving the eyes downward.
- **CN V: Trigeminal:** Face feeling & chewing nerve. Facial pain, numbness, tingling, or altered sensation in the forehead, cheek, or jaw.
- **CN VI: Abducens:** Eye side-movement nerve. Inability to move the eye outward, causing horizontal double vision.

- **CN VII: Facial:** Face movement and front of tongue nerve. Facial weakness or asymmetry, drooling, dry eye, or altered taste on the front of the tongue.
- **CN VIII: Vestibulocochlear:** Hearing and balance nerve. Hearing loss, tinnitus, balance issues, or vertigo.
- **CN IX: Glossopharyngeal:** Tongue and throat nerve. Difficulty swallowing, sore throat, or loss of taste in the back of the tongue.
- **CN X: Vagus:** From the Latin word "to wander". The nerve from the brain to the gut. Hoarseness, swallowing difficulties, irregular heart rate, nausea, gastrointestinal symptoms etc.
- **CN XI: Accessory:** Neck and shoulder movement nerve. Weakness in shoulder elevation or head rotation.
- **CN XII: Hypoglossal:** Tongue movement nerve. Tongue weakness, slurred speech, or difficulty swallowing.

Other Possible Radiologic Findings

Although more research is needed to fully understand craniocervical instability, there are several conditions that may be commonly seen alongside it. The following list includes possible findings that can appear on imaging studies when there are abnormal findings at the craniocervical junction. Keep in mind that not all of these conditions will apply to every patient, as each case is unique.

This list serves as a general guide to some of the conditions that *might* be seen in patients with craniocervical instability:

- Scoliosis and Kyphosis
- Platybasia
- Syringomyelia / Syrinx
- Retroflexed Odontoid
- Tarlov Cysts
- Other damage, injury and degeneration etc.

***Note:** Not all patients with CCI will have these findings, and the presence or significance of each can vary widely. This list is a collection of potential comorbidities, but these are not exclusive to CCI and may not have a clear causative relationship in every case.

Tethered Cord Syndrome

Tethered cord syndrome (TCS) is a condition that *may* occur alongside craniocervical instability, however more research is necessary. If left undiagnosed, it may lead to complications, especially if spinal surgery like craniocervical fusion surgery is planned.

To detect this difficult to identify condition, a specialized lumbar MRI is done in the supine (lying on back) and sometimes prone position (lying on the stomach); although the use of prone MRI as a standard for diagnosing tethered cord is not part of mainstream protocols at this time. It is also important to note that tethered cord syndrome (TCS) can be occult, meaning it is hidden or not seen on imaging.

A supine and/or prone MRI of the lumbosacral spine allows radiologists to closely examine the lower spinal cord and surrounding structures. In the MRI, radiologists check for key signs of tethered cord syndrome, such as:

- A low-lying conus medullaris (the end of the spinal cord sitting lower than normal)
- Thickening of the filum (greater than 2mm)
- Fat in the filum terminale (a small cord at the base of the spine)
- The terminal filum shows restricted or absent movement
- Restricted conus mobility
- In prone position, the terminal filum is separated from the cauda equina and is shifted caudally to posteriorly in the subarachnoid space. *Note: This displacement is not a widely recognized standard MRI finding or diagnostic criterion; and at this time lacks broad peer-reviewed support.

A low-lying conus medullaris, thickened or fatty filum terminale, and limited mobility of the cord/filum are well-documented criteria.

The prone position axial MRI, also known as Prone Position Testing (PPT) and the Kazuyoshi Protocol, are the prone MRI imaging tethered cord protocols, that add important information by showing how the spinal cord and filum behave when the body is in a different position. This can reveal subtle signs of tethering or abnormal stretching that might not appear in the supine scan.

Key Decision Factor #3 - Failure of Conservative Treatments

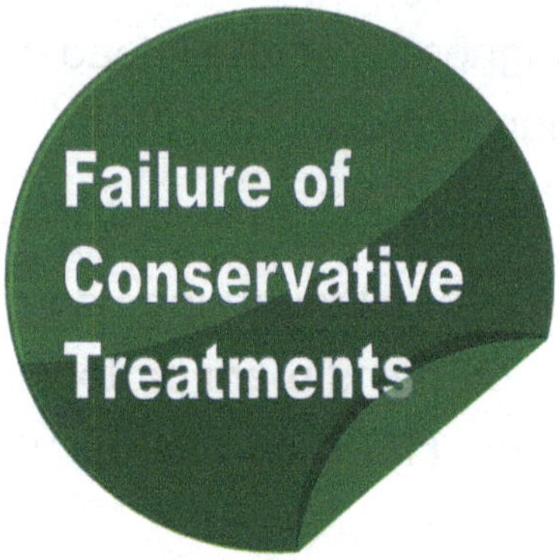

If a patient has been following a consistent conservative (non-surgical) treatment plan for non-urgent craniocervical instability for 6 months without improvement, it may be time to consult a neurosurgeon. This is especially true if neurological symptoms do not improve. Conservative care options may include but are not limited to:

- pacing, a self-management strategy for activity.

- upper cervical chiropractic treatments

- physiotherapy interventions such as:

  - relief of muscle tension, for example, in the upper trapezius, sternocleidomastoid (SCM) and suboccipital muscles through targeted techniques that reduce pain and restore proper function;

  - a neuro-oriented PT that focuses on head/neck proprioception, balance, and gentle stabilization; and

  - cervical stabilization exercises to improve strength of deep neck flexors, postural and core muscles; or vestibular rehabilitation if dizziness or balance is affected.

- medications, topical agents and/or supplements for pain management

- fluoroscopy-guided injections like platelet-rich plasma (although more studies are needed to prove its effectiveness), occipital nerve blocks and cervical medial branch blocks

- Wearing a neck / cervical bracing with a soft or hard collar when doing specific tasks to avoid neck movements or flexion (but not often to avoid muscle atrophy/weakening

- ergonomic supports and postural modifications such as reducing movements or head positions that aggravate symptoms, a supportive chair, keeping neck in neutral position, spine neutral sleeping positions, adjustable beds (elevated head-of-bed sleeping (30–45°), cervical pillows, using grabber tools etc.

- craniosacral therapy, cognitive behavioral therapy, stress reduction techniques such as slow breathing or mindfulness

- anti-inflammatory diet, hydration and salt & sugar restriction

- vagus nerve stimulation
- lymphatic drainage
- platelet rich plasma (PRP) or other orthobiological fluoroscopy guided injections
- other as directed by a treating healthcare provider.

While there is no exact timeline, many neurosurgeons suggest seeking a surgical opinion after about six months of unsuccessful conservative treatment. Surgery is usually not the first option and is typically reserved for cases where symptoms are severe, life-threatening, or do not respond to conservative treatments.

Since each patient's case is different and there is limited research on the best conservative treatments and their duration, it is important to work closely with healthcare providers specializing in the upper cervical spine.

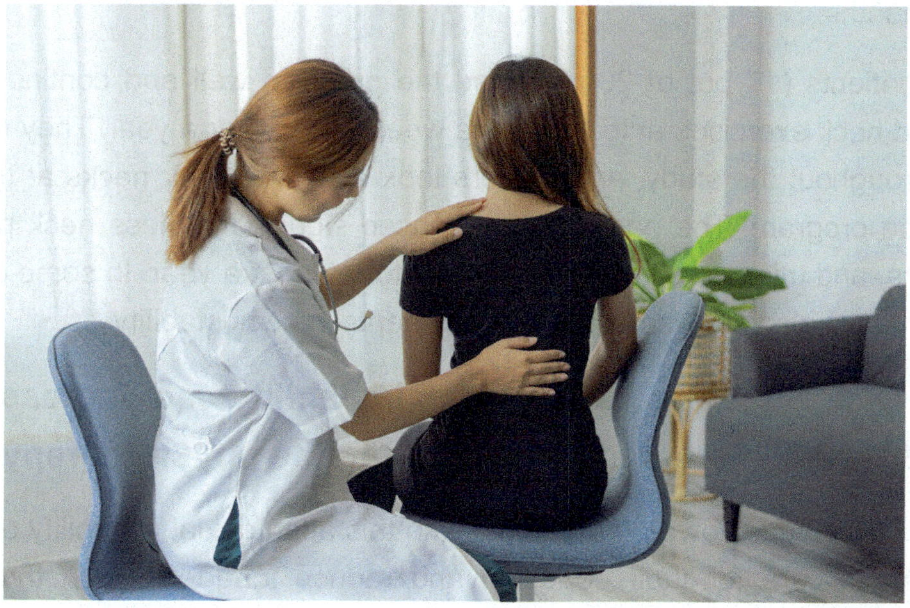

Physiotherapy May Reduce Atlantoaxial Instability

In a 1998 study, twenty people with atlantoaxial instability (i.e., the joint is too loose or moves too much and can't stay in the correct position) caused by *rheumatoid arthritis* took part in a non-surgical treatment program. The goal was to reduce their symptoms and slow the progression of their condition. The treatment lasted two weeks in the hospital and involved support from a team of health professionals. The program included several parts: patient education, physiotherapy, use of neck collars, practical tools for daily living, treatments to relieve symptoms, and medications that target the underlying (rheumatic) disease.

Patients were taught about the anatomy of the neck area of the spine. A key point emphasized was that bending the neck forward (flexion) and turning the neck (rotation) is harmful to people with unstable atlantoaxial joints and should be avoided. Patients also received training in proper body mechanics and ergonomics.

The researchers concluded that it is possible to educate and motivate people with atlantoaxial instability or subluxation to take an active role in caring for their necks. This can help relieve chronic neck pain and may even slow the progression of arthritis in the cervical spine. The goal was to prevent complications and reduce the need for surgery. After the hospital stay, patients continued the program at home and returned for checkups at 6 and 12 months.

Most of the patients (17 out of 20) followed the program well and continued doing the recommended neck exercises at least once a week, even after a year. They reported their symptoms throughout the study, and doctors took X-rays of their necks at the beginning and end of the program. The patients experienced significantly less neck pain after the first two weeks, and this improvement continued for at least a year. In some cases, the X-rays also showed small improvements in neck stability.

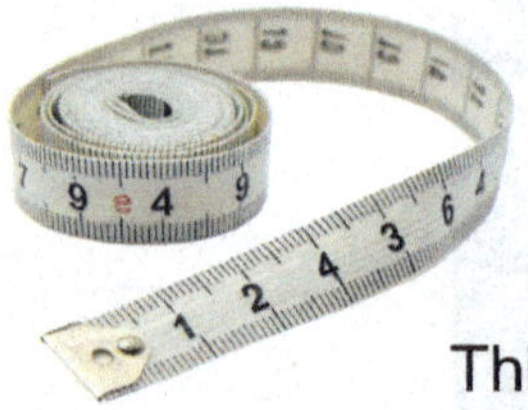

In three patients, the instability had decreased by 3 millimeters after completing the physiotherapy program.

This study showed that people with this atlantoaxial instability or subluxation can learn to care for their condition and reduce long-term pain through regular exercise and proper support. In some cases, the instability in the neck may also improve without surgery.

Managing Craniocervical Instability in Hypermobility and Ehlers-Danlos Syndrome

For some people with craniocervical instability caused by conditions like generalized joint hypermobility or Ehlers-Danlos syndrome, mild symptoms can often be managed with pain relief and physical therapy. However, more serious cases may need the guidance of a neurosurgeon.

Important Note: Before starting any physical therapy, it is very important for patients to complete imaging studies like a dynamic upright MRI and dynamic CT scan or uCBCT scan. Once the tests are completed, patients should bring the reports to both their doctor and physical therapist. The doctor must confirm that it is safe for patients to begin therapy.

To help improve treatment for this condition, a team of physical therapists with experience in craniocervical instability and a rheumatologist who specializes in joint hypermobility worked together to create new guidelines. They developed a system to help identify how severe and reactive each person's symptoms may be. This is called "mechanical irritability" of the CCJ. **Mechanical irritability refers to how easily symptoms are triggered by movement, how intense the symptoms are, and how long they last after a flare-up.**

There are three levels of irritability: low, moderate, and high. People with low irritability usually have symptoms that stay steady and are not easily triggered. People with moderate irritability may have occasional flare-ups, but they recover in a reasonable amount of time. People with high irritability have very sensitive symptoms. Even small movements or changes can cause strong symptoms that take a long time to settle. These individuals may need to use a wheelchair, spend most of their time in bed, or avoid certain activities completely.

Experts recommend that patients see a neurosurgeon if they have a high level of mechanical irritability that prevents them from starting or continuing physical therapy. A referral is also important if symptoms are getting worse over time or are not improving with rest, medication, and regular therapy. Some warning signs that may mean the patient urgently needs to see a neurosurgeon include drop attacks, fainting with neck movement, seizure-like episodes, choking, voice changes, trouble swallowing, or severe problems with vision and balance. If patients cannot stay upright without symptoms getting worse, or if their doctor suspects vertical instability in the upper part of the neck, a neurosurgeon should be involved early.

Even though there are no official guidelines, many doctors agree that when vertical instability is suspected, it is safest to have a neurosurgeon approve the therapy plan before beginning physical treatment. In less severe cases, a neurosurgeon may recommend trying physical therapy for up to six months before considering surgery.

Treatment plans depend on how irritable the condition is. Patients are grouped into low, moderate, or high irritability categories, and each group has different recommendations. For all patients, education is one of the most important parts of care. This includes learning about posture, safe body movements, how to complete daily tasks with less strain, and how to manage pain. A neck brace may be helpful during flare-ups, while traveling, or while waiting for a surgical consultation. Relaxation techniques like slow breathing or mindfulness can also help reduce pain sensitivity.

High Irritability

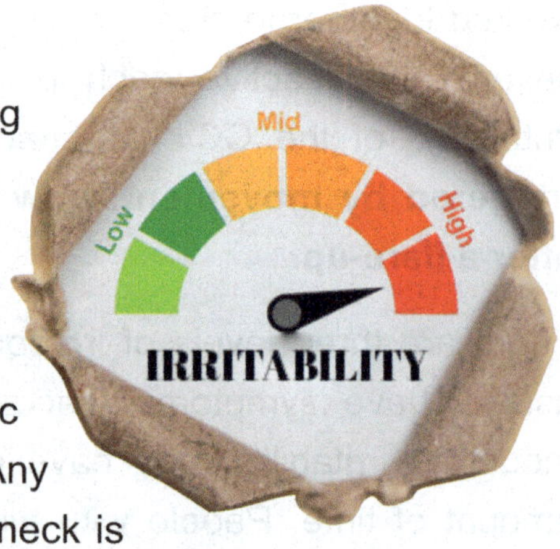

For patients with high irritability, the focus is on avoiding flare-ups. Many of these individuals cannot tolerate physical exercises or manual therapy. Instead, therapy focuses on education, resting positions, and bracing. If tolerated, very gentle movements in supported positions may be introduced, along with light aerobic activities like a recumbent bike or walking in water. Any exercise or treatment that could place pressure on the neck is avoided.

Moderate Irritability

For patients with moderate irritability, therapy can include gentle strength exercises and movement control training. This includes working on the legs, shoulders, and spine, along with light neck training that avoids any sudden or large movements. Walking and stationary cycling may also be included. Manual therapy is allowed only if the therapist is well-trained.

Low Irritability

For patients with low irritability, therapy can be more advanced. They may be able to participate in posture training, light core strengthening, and gradual neck movements. However, aggressive neck manipulations should still be avoided.

Finding the Right Physical Therapist

Because CCI is complex and not widely understood, it is important to find a physical therapist who has experience with joint hypermobility, EDS and upper cervical instability, or a PT who is open and willing to learn. Some therapists may not fully understand how delicate these conditions can be. Using the wrong exercises could make symptoms worse. A book, *Living Life to the Fullest with Ehlers-Danilo's Syndrome* by Kathleen and Kevin Muldowney is a guide for both the physiotherapist and patients with EDS (and can be used by non-EDS patients with CCI).

If a patient's symptoms have not improved after attending physical therapy two or three times per week for about six months, or if they are unsure whether it is safe to begin therapy at all, patients should speak with their doctor about seeing a neurosurgeon. While many people with this condition can improve without surgery, others may need help from a specialist to find the best path forward.

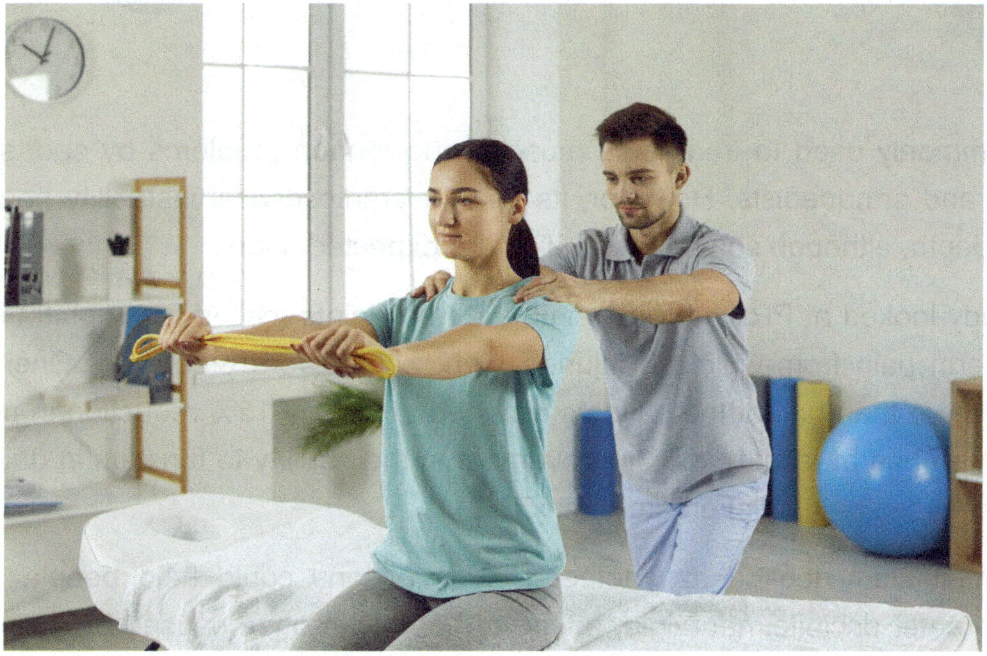

Platelet-Rich Plasma Injections

Platelet-rich plasma (PRP) therapy is a treatment that uses a patient's own blood to help promote healing. Blood is made up of different parts, including red blood cells, white blood cells, and platelets. Platelets are tiny cell fragments that help with clotting and contain growth factors that support tissue repair. In PRP therapy, the patient's blood is processed to concentrate the platelets, and this platelet-rich mixture is then injected into injured or painful areas of the body.

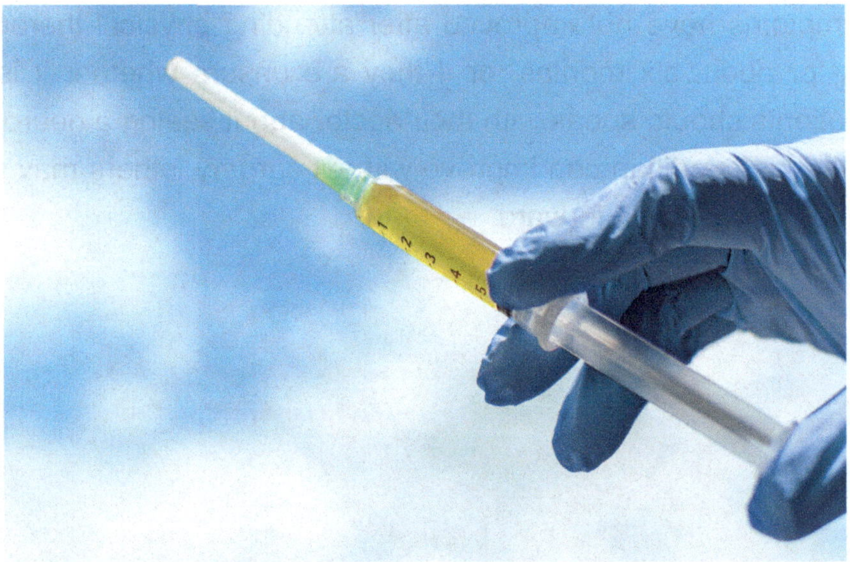

PRP is commonly used to treat joint, muscle, and tendon problems by sports medicine specialists and orthopedists. However, its use for craniocervical instability has not been studied in depth, although some new studies are expected soon.

A 2023 study looked at PRP injections into the neck joints (called facet joints) in patients with long-term pain from whiplash injuries. The results were promising. One year after treatment, more than half of the patients reported at least a 15% reduction in pain. About 70% said they had at least a 10% improvement in their ability to function in daily life, and some experienced pain relief greater than 50%.

A 2024 small study looked at whether PRP injections could help people with post-traumatic greater occipital neuralgia, a type of headache often caused by injury. Patients were given either PRP, a steroid/anesthetic mix, or a saltwater (saline) injection. PRP showed some improvements in how headaches affected daily life after 3 months, but there was no clear difference in pain levels between the groups. The researchers concluded that more studies are needed.

A small 2021 study followed 14 patients with long-term neck pain who received regenerative injections instead of relying on medications or surgery. Each person was treated with a combination of platelet-rich plasma, platelet lysate, and prolotherapy (natural substances made from the patient's own blood to promote healing). A trained physician used fluoroscopy (real-time X-ray) to guide the injections into neck joints, ligaments, and near nerves. Most patients received one treatment and were followed for two years. Most saw significant improvements in pain and function.

These results suggest PRP may help with certain neck-related conditions. However, since the studies focused on whiplash injuries and post-traumatic greater occipital neuralgia, neck pain and not specifically craniocervical instability, it is not yet clear if the same benefits would apply.

Research is needed to understand how effective PRP is for craniocervical instability. Patients considering PRP therapy for craniocervical instability should speak with a healthcare provider who specializes in PRP for upper cervical spinal disorders.

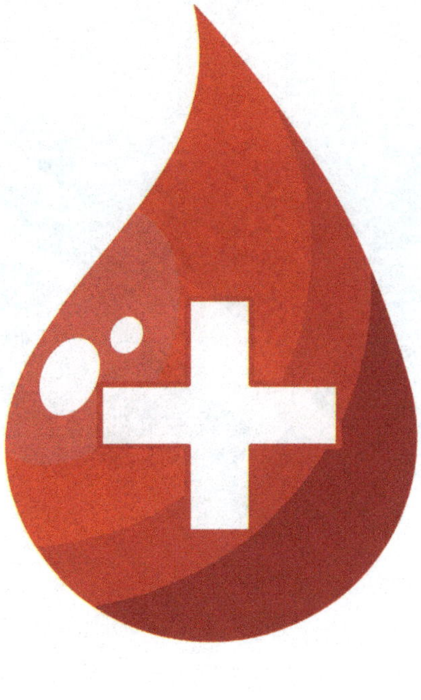

PICL: Investigational Regenerative Injection for Craniocervical Instability (Under Clinical Trial)

Percutaneous Implantation of Craniocervical Ligaments (PICL) is a specialized, non-surgical procedure developed by Dr. Chris Centeno at the Centeno-Schultz Clinic in Colorado, USA, for treating craniocervical instability. PICL involves injecting orthobiologics (such as bone marrow concentrate and PRP) into the damaged ligaments at the base of the skull and upper cervical spine through the mouth using precise fluoroscopic guidance.

While the procedure is only available at this clinic, a randomized controlled trial (RCT) including a placebo (sham) group is currently underway to evaluate its safety and effectiveness. As of now, no peer-reviewed studies on PICL have been published, but the clinic reports that a case series with imaging outcomes is in preparation. Dr. Centeno has authored numerous peer-reviewed articles on orthobiologics, regenerative spine and joint therapies, and image-guided injection techniques. PICL may offer promising treatment for CCI patients not offered or wanting to avoid fusion surgery.

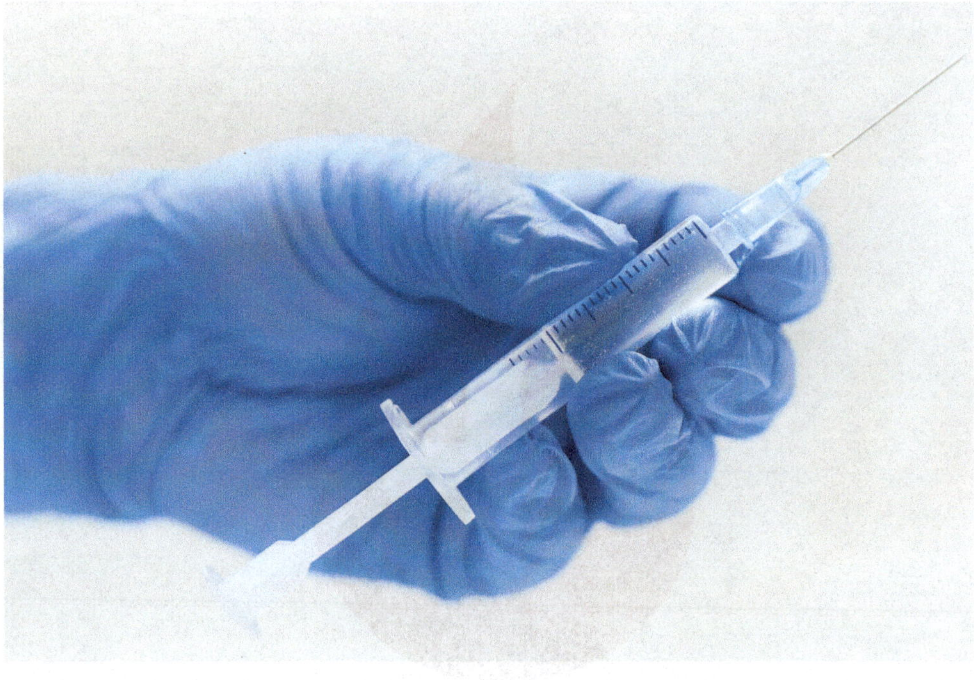

Soft Neck Brace with or without Jaw Support

A soft cervical collar with jaw support is a medical device designed to stabilize the neck and head and may especially be helpful for conditions like craniocervical instability. These collars are usually made from soft foam and have chin support to limit head movement and reduce pain.

To choose the right size, measure the neck circumference or follow the sizing guides provided by the manufacturer. Look for breathable, hypoallergenic materials to avoid skin irritation. Collars that include chin and jaw support may provide better stability. Wear the collar as advised by a healthcare provider, during specific activities and perhaps while sleeping.

Patients should always consult their healthcare provider before using a cervical collar. Long-term use can have negative effects and make the neck muscles weak, worsening craniocervical instability due to muscle weakness.

A soft collar with jaw support may offer improved stabilization for some patients, though it can be uncomfortable or exacerbate pain; in such cases, transitioning to a soft collar without jaw support may be more tolerable.

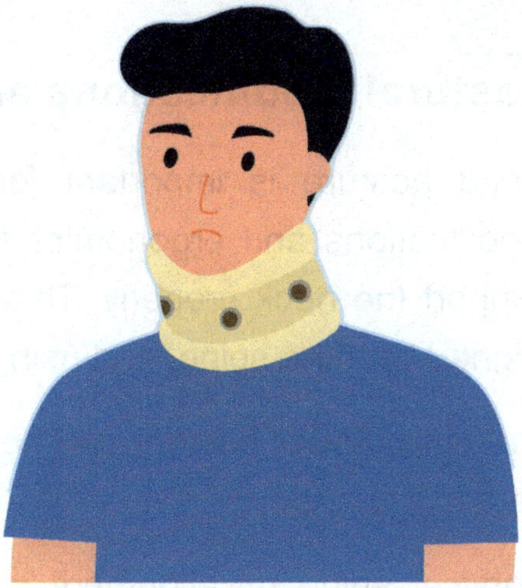

If any type of collar causes significant discomfort, patients are advised to consult with their physiotherapist or specialist to explore alternative options.

If a cervical brace is uncomfortable, a physiotherapist may adjust its fit for better support, recommend gentle neck mobility and stretching exercises to reduce stiffness, apply soft tissue techniques to relieve muscle tension (such as the upper trapezius, sternocleidomastoid, and suboccipital muscles), and suggest alternative support options to improve comfort while maintaining proper neck alignment.

In more severe cases, healthcare providers may recommend the use of a hard cervical collar to provide greater stability. Although a cervical collar may be a useful conservative treatment device for a short period of time, research has shown that wearing one for an extended period of time may lead to weakening and stiffening of the neck muscles.

Heat and Cold Therapy

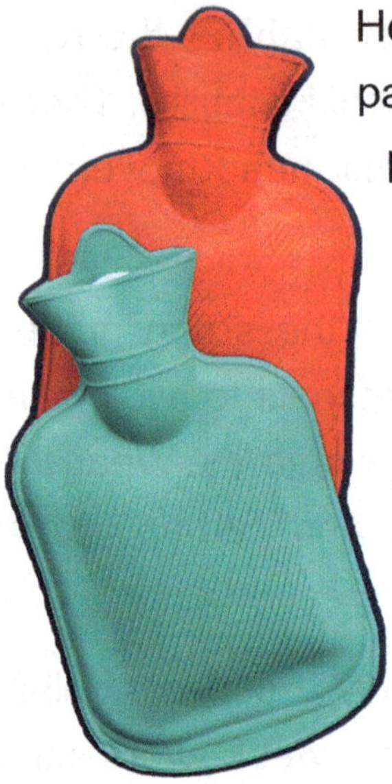

Heat and cold therapy involve using hot or cold packs to help manage pain and reduce swelling. Both treatments are easy to use and can provide relief from neck pain. Always use a barrier, like a towel, to protect the skin from direct contact with the pack.

- **Cold packs** can numb the area, decrease inflammation, and ease muscle pain.
- **Heat packs** help increase blood flow, relax muscles, and soothe stiffness.

Postural Modifications and Ergonomics

Good posture is important for reducing neck strain during daily activities. Postural modifications and ergonomics teach patients how to sit, stand, and move in ways that support the neck properly. This includes sitting with the back straight, keeping the head aligned with the spine, and using chairs or tools that support the body's natural position.

Learning proper posture can help prevent neck pain and improve comfort throughout the day.

Cervical spine misalignment correlates with higher pain intensity and disability levels. Studies have shown that maintaining a neutral cervical spine alignment can significantly reduce neck pain and improve function. Research indicates that individuals with forward head posture often experience increased neck pain and disability.

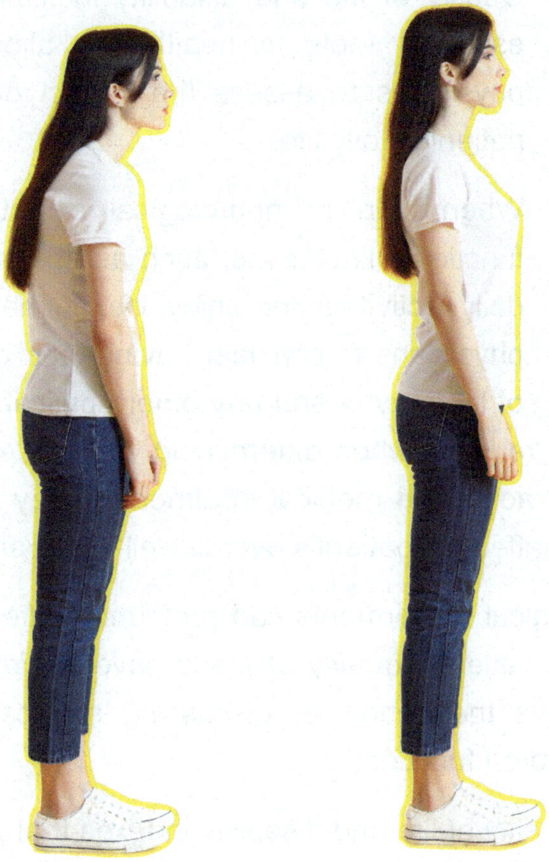

Other Conservative Treatments

While this overview has introduced some of the commonly recommended conservative treatments, it's important to note that other options such as osteopathic (OMP) treatments provided by a Doctor of Osteopathic Medicine (DO) exist and can be very helpful. However, covering all available treatments in detail would go beyond the scope of this chapter. The goal here is to provide a basic understanding of typical first-line recommendations, but patients should be aware that additional therapies may be appropriate depending on their condition and specialist guidance.

Key Decision Factor #4 - Quality of Life and Disability Indices

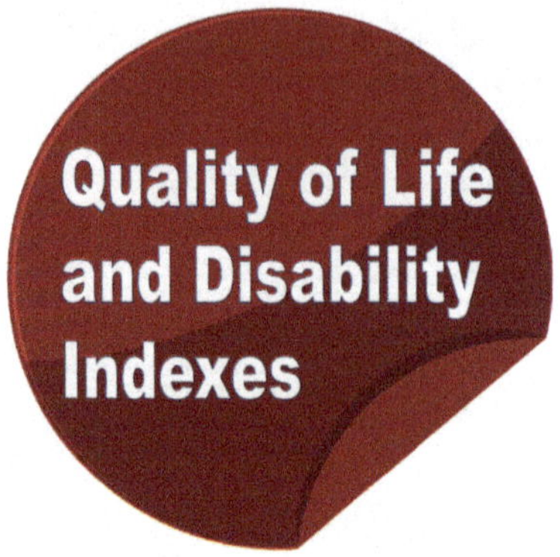

Quality of life and disability indices and questionnaires are essential tools in healthcare, allowing both patients and physicians to assess the impact of health conditions on a patient's daily life.

When pain or neurological symptoms lead to significant functional limitations, such as an inability to work, engage in daily activities, or enjoy life, it may be crucial for treating physicians to consider having their patient complete a quality of life survey and any other applicable questionnaires. These measures are particularly valuable when determining whether a patient should consult a neurosurgeon or consider advanced medical treatments. They provide a structured way to assess how a condition affects a patient's overall well-being and daily functioning.

Chronic pain and neurological impairments can profoundly affect a patient's mental and emotional well-being. If a patient's *quality of life* is severely impacted and non-surgical treatments do not improve the condition, discussing surgical options may offer the potential for relief and restored function.

The following are some quality of life and disability indexes that patients can use, keeping in mind they do not have to do all of them, and it is best to talk to their healthcare providers to discuss which ones would be most relevant.

Note: Quality of life and disability indices that have been developed and validated through clinical research can provide objective evidence that can support insurance or legal claims. While these indices alone don't prove disability, they are valuable when combined with medical evaluations, helping to demonstrate the real-life impact of a condition on work and daily activities. When properly ordered and validated by a physician, particularly a reputable specialist, they can also serve as supporting evidence in insurance claims to help demonstrate disability based on policy criteria, such as inability to perform one's own job, any job, or meeting the threshold for programs that define disability as severe and permanent.

Quality of Life (QoL)

Quality of Life (QoL) refers to a patient’s general well-being, encompassing physical, emotional, social, and functional health. Healthcare professionals use various QoL assessments to gain insight into how a condition and its treatment affect a patient's everyday activities.

A commonly used tool for measuring quality of life in clinical practice is the **Short Form 36 (SF-36)**, a survey of 36 questions that evaluates a range of health aspects, including physical functioning, bodily pain, general health, vitality, and emotional well-being.

Specialists such as primary care physicians, orthopaedic surgeons, neurologists, pain specialists, and oncologists often use this tool to understand the broad impact of a condition on a patient’s life. Surgery may be considered when the results of the SF-36 survey indicate significant limitations in key areas such as physical functioning, bodily pain, or general health.

Specifically, if the survey shows severe or very severe limitations, such as high pain levels, inability to perform daily activities, or reduced overall well-being, surgery may be considered as a potential option to improve quality of life. However, the decision also depends on factors such as the specific condition, its prognosis, and the patient's overall health.

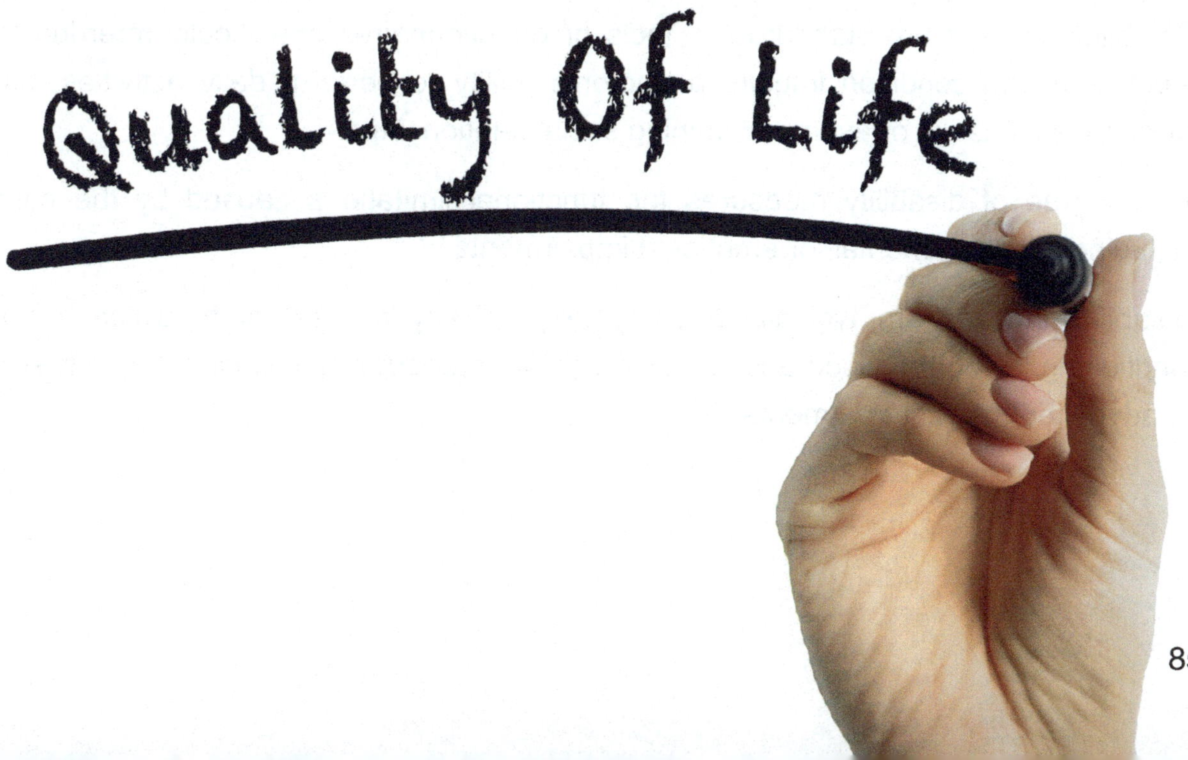

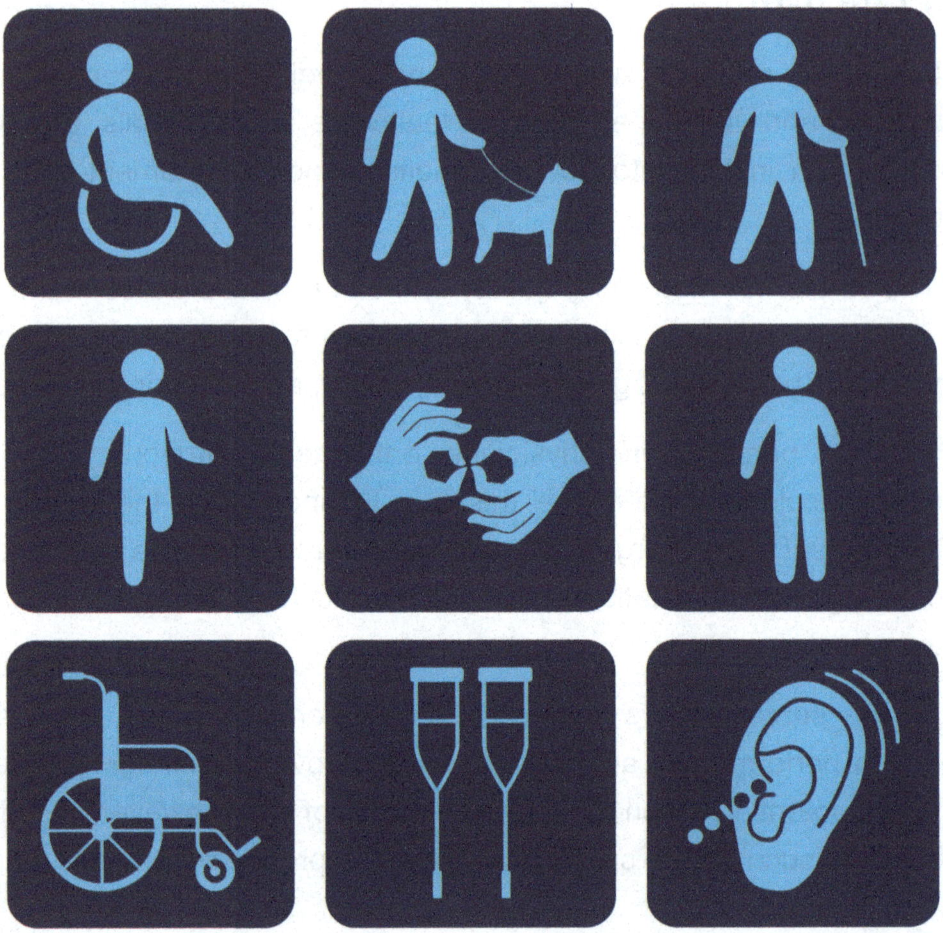

Disability Indexes

Disability indexes are standardized tools or questionnaires specifically referring to how much a health condition impairs a person's ability to perform daily activities, such as working, exercising, or even maintaining social relationships.

The degree of disability measures the functional limitations caused by the condition, including physical, mental, or emotional impairments.

Disability indexes are typically used to help identify the extent to which a patient's functioning is compromised and to guide decisions about rehabilitation, support services, or advanced medical treatments.

Neck Disability Index

The Neck Disability Index (NDI) is a widely used self-reported questionnaire that assesses how neck pain impacts daily activities. It includes 10 items covering areas such as pain, personal care, work, sleep, and recreation.

Commonly used for conditions like chronic neck pain, whiplash, and cervical radiculopathy, the NDI helps track symptom severity and treatment progress. While generally reliable, its accuracy can vary based on patient condition and test administration.

Moderate to severe scores often guide clinicians toward more intensive treatments, including surgery, particularly when conservative approaches fail to provide relief.

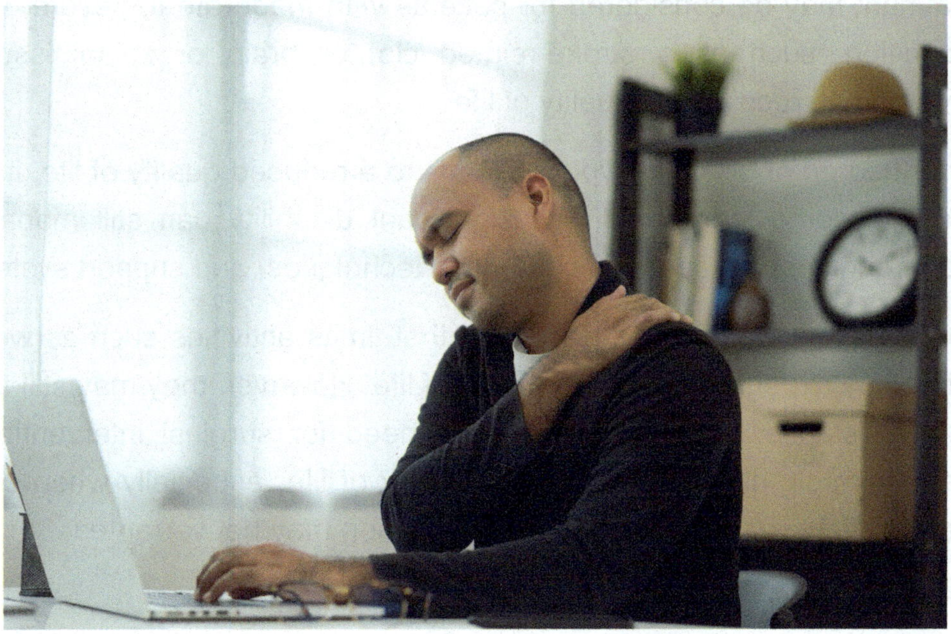

Modified Rankin Scale

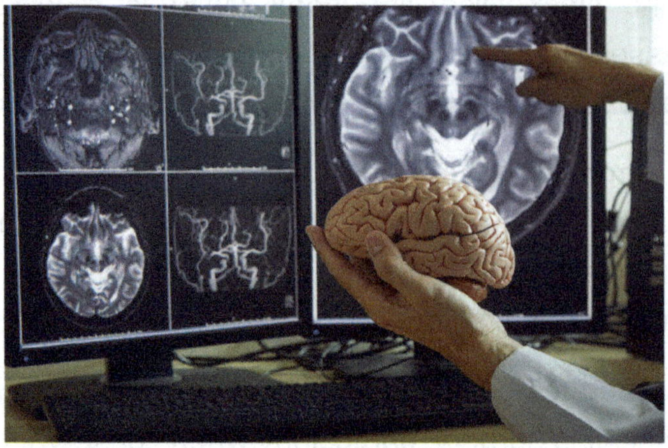

The Modified Rankin Scale (mRS) is a gold-standard tool used for assessing disability following stroke, cerebrovascular events, or neurological conditions, though its relevance to craniocervical instability may be limited.

The mRS works by assessing a patient's level of disability or dependence based on their ability to perform daily activities.

After a stroke or neurological event, healthcare providers use the mRS to assess the level of assistance a patient requires in daily activities. mRS helps healthcare providers track recovery or progression, as well as guide treatment decisions.

Surgical treatment may be considered for patients with moderate to severe disability if a treatable condition, such as a stroke-related clot or brain or spinal issue, can be addressed to improve recovery or quality of life.

While a higher degree of disability typically leads to a reduced quality of life, it's important to recognize that some individuals with significant disability can still manage a good quality of life through coping strategies, adaptive techniques, and support systems.

For example, a patient with severe neck pain that limits activities such as work, driving, and recreation may experience a lower quality of life. However, they may still find ways to function with assistance, which can delay the need for surgical intervention. If these symptoms are severely affecting a patient's quality of life, especially when conservative treatments are ineffective, a neurosurgical consultation may be warranted.

Karnofsky Performance Scale (KPS)

The Karnofsky Performance Scale (KPS) is another helpful medical tool for measuring the degree of disability, particularly in assessing a patient's ability to perform daily activities and self-care. It is commonly used in oncology, palliative care and other medical fields to evaluate the impact of a disease on a patient's overall function and quality of life. A lower score on the Karnofsky Scale often indicates a reduced quality of life, as a person with more disability may experience greater challenges in daily living, social interactions, and overall happiness.

Karnofsky Scale Scoring System:

The scale ranges from 0 to 100, with higher scores indicating better performance and functional status.

100: Normal, no complaints; no evidence of disease

90: Able to carry on normal activity; minor signs or symptoms of disease

80: Normal activity with effort; some symptoms of disease

70: Cares for self; unable to carry on normal activity or to do active work. (Patient is able to independently care for themselves but struggles with work or strenuous activities).

60: Requires occasional assistance but is able to care for most of their needs. (Patient is mostly independent but may need some help with certain tasks due to moderate symptoms or physical limitations).

50: Requires considerable assistance and frequent medical care. (Patient can perform only some basic activities and needs regular help for day-to-day tasks).

40: Disabled; requires special care and assistance. (Patient is largely bedridden, requiring help with most daily activities).

30: Severely disabled; hospitalization is indicated, although death is not imminent

20: Very sick; hospital admission necessary; active supportive treatment is needed

10: Moribund; fatal processes progressing rapidly (near death)

0: Dead

EQ-5D Health-Related Quality of Life Questionnaire

The EuroQol-5D (EQ-5D) is a widely used health-related quality of life measure that provides a simple, short, standardized way to assess a patient's overall health status. It evaluates five key dimensions of health: mobility, self-care, usual activities, pain/discomfort, and anxiety/depression.

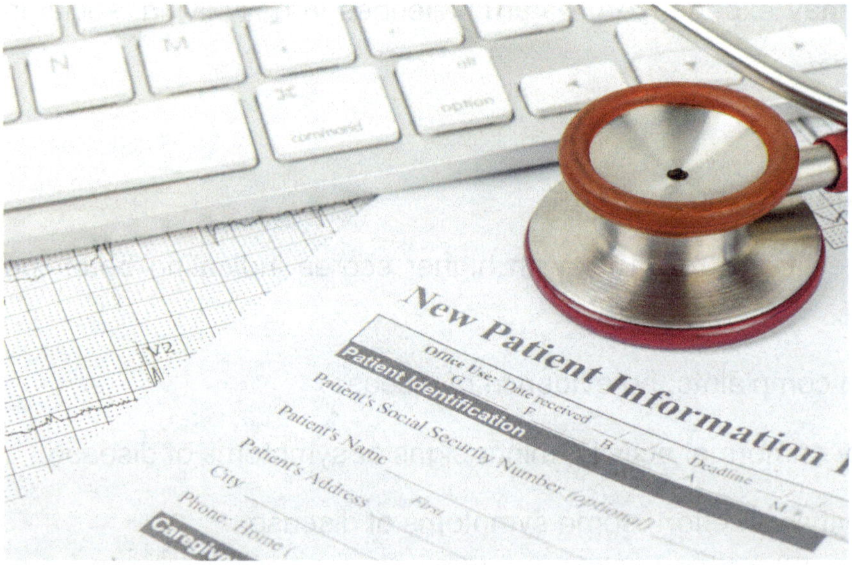

Each dimension is rated on a scale from no problems to extreme problems, allowing healthcare providers to capture a quick snapshot of a patient's functional status.

It can be a valuable tool for assessing how the condition impacts a patient's daily life. The measure is reliable in reflecting changes in health status over time, making it useful for tracking the progression of symptoms.

If the results indicate significant impairment in health-related quality of life, it may be time to consult with a neurosurgeon.

Study: Before and After Craniocervical Fusion Surgery - A EuroQol-5D Study on Quality of Life

A study led from Pomeranian Medical University in Poland explored how patients with craniocervical instability felt before and after undergoing spinal surgery. The research followed 60 patients who had surgery to stabilize the upper spine using the Goel-Harms technique. This is a common method where screws are inserted into the top two bones of the spine (C1 and C2) and connected with rods to keep the bones in place. Some patients also had a plate attached to the back of the skull to provide extra support, depending on how unstable their condition was.

To assess how the patients felt, the team used the quality of life survey EQ-5D, which is designed to measure various aspects of a person's health. The survey asks about pain, mobility, self-care, usual activities, and anxiety or depression. Patients completed this survey both before their surgery and about two years after the surgery.

Before surgery, the average quality of life score for the patients was 0.254, reflecting a very poor quality of life. This score is on a scale where 1 means perfect health, and 0 means the worst possible health (equivalent to death). Most patients reported significant difficulty with pain, movement, and performing daily activities. Many also experienced high levels of anxiety or depression.

After surgery, there was a significant improvement in the patients' quality of life (QoL). Their average score increased to 0.779, showing that the surgery helped to reduce pain, improve movement, and enhance mental health. However, even after two years, their scores were still lower than the average quality of life score of people without CCI, which is around 0.894.

RESULTS BASED ON EUROQOL-5D QUALITY OF LIFE SCORES

1.0 = Perfect Health

Before Surgery Average Score	After Surgery Average Score	Population Average Score
0.254	0.779	0.894

The study also revealed that adding a skull plate to the surgery (called occipital plating) did not make a significant difference in the long-term health outcomes. Patients with and without the plate showed similar improvements in their quality of life after surgery. This finding helps clarify an ongoing debate in spinal surgery about the importance of this extra support.

The study found that younger patients tended to recover better than older patients. Older patients often experienced less improvement in their health after surgery. The reason for this could be slower healing, additional health problems, or reduced mobility in older age. Another important factor was the length of hospital stay. Patients who spent more time in the hospital had worse outcomes, which could indicate complications like infections or slower recovery processes.

Imaging tests, particularly a measurement called the Wackenheim line (used to assess the alignment of the spine), were also examined in the study. Some patients with abnormal measurements of this line had worse recovery outcomes, but the link wasn't strong enough to be used as a reliable predictor for recovery.

One of the most significant improvements after surgery was in pain and mental health. Before surgery, almost all patients reported moderate to severe pain and high levels of anxiety or depression. After the surgery, these issues improved the most. Pain levels were reduced, and mental health generally improved, helping patients feel better overall. However, some patients, particularly older individuals, continued to have trouble with daily activities and self-care even after the surgery.

The EQ-5D questionnaire is designed to measure five key dimensions of health: mobility, self-care, usual activities, pain/discomfort, and anxiety/depression. These dimensions give a clear picture of a patient's overall quality of life.

- **Mobility:** Before surgery, most patients reported severe issues with mobility, often having difficulty walking or moving around due to pain and instability in the spine. The surgery led to significant improvements in this area, with many patients reporting that they could move with less discomfort and more ease two years after surgery. The average improvement in this category was substantial, with patients moving from a state of severe problems to moderate or mild issues.
- **Self-Care:** Prior to surgery, many patients struggled with basic tasks like dressing, bathing, and eating, due to the limitations caused by their condition. After surgery, most patients reported improvements in their ability to perform self-care tasks

independently, although some older patients still had difficulty. The overall score for self-care improved significantly after surgery, indicating that patients could better manage their personal hygiene and daily tasks.

- **Usual Activities:** Before surgery, many patients were unable to participate in normal daily activities like work, hobbies, or social interactions due to pain and mobility issues. After the surgery, there was a noticeable improvement in this dimension, though full recovery to a normal level of activity was not achieved by all. Younger patients showed more dramatic improvements in resuming their usual activities compared to older patients.

- **Pain/Discomfort:** This was one of the most improved categories. Before surgery, nearly all patients experienced moderate to severe pain. After surgery, pain was significantly reduced for most patients, improving their overall quality of life. The reduction in pain was a key factor in the increase in overall health scores.

- **Anxiety/Depression:** Patients reported high levels of anxiety and depression before surgery. After surgery, many patients felt less anxious and depressed, as their physical function improved, and they regained more independence. This was another major contributor to the improved overall quality of life scores.

This study highlights that the Goel-Harms technique for stabilizing the upper spine in patients with craniocervical instability can significantly improve quality of life. While surgery leads to improvements in mobility, pain, and mental health, full recovery to normal levels is difficult to achieve, especially for older patients or those with longer hospital stays. The study also suggests that the addition of a skull plate does not provide significant additional benefits in improving the patient's quality of life, which could help simplify the decision-making process for doctors and patients when considering surgery.

Overall, the findings from the EuroQol-5D survey show that surgical treatment for CCI helps patients feel much better but doesn't always return them to the health levels of the general population. This study is important as it gives doctors and patients a clearer understanding of what they may expect after surgery and helps them make better-informed decisions about treatment options.

Montreal Cognitive Assessment

The Montreal Cognitive Assessment (MoCA) is a standardized screening tool used to assess a patient's cognitive function, evaluating areas such as memory, attention, language, executive function, visuospatial abilities, and orientation.

It is widely regarded for its reliability in detecting mild cognitive impairment and is often used in clinical settings to monitor cognitive changes over time.

The MoCA can be an important diagnostic tool to identify subtle cognitive deficits that may result from compression of neural structures.

Given its sensitivity in detecting early cognitive decline, the MoCA can help physicians gauge the impact of CCI on cognitive function. If results indicate significant cognitive impairment, further evaluation by a neurosurgeon is warranted.

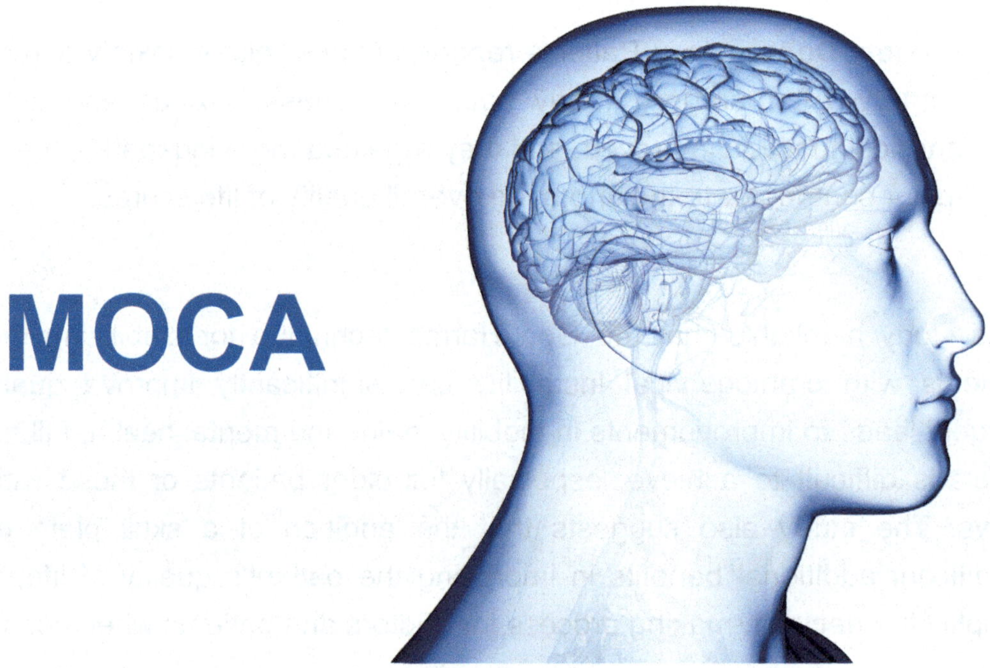

Patient Health Questionnaire (PHQ-9) and Generalized Anxiety Disorder (GAD-7)

The PHQ-9 and GAD-7 are simple questionnaires that help doctors understand how much someone is experiencing symptoms of depression and anxiety. They ask about mood, worry, energy, and daily functioning to guide care and treatment. Both are well-validated, reliable clinical tools.

Key Decision Factor #5 - Patient-Specific Factors

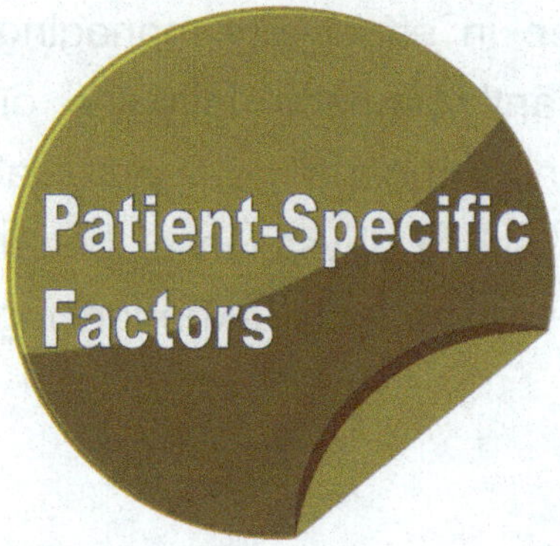

Age, Health, Risks

Overall health plays a significant role in determining the risks and benefits of surgery, especially those that smoke, are obese, or have significant comorbidities. The age of the patient also plays a key factor in determining the risks and benefits of surgery.

In general, patients that are older, who smoke or are obese or have significant comorbidities may face different surgical risks compared to other patients. A neurosurgeon can assess whether the potential benefits of surgery outweigh the risks based on the patient's age, overall health, and specific condition(s).

Seeking the opinion of a neurosurgeon specializing in craniocervical instability can help confirm whether spine conditions are contributing to their symptoms and offer clarity on surgical options.

The Role of Peace of Mind in Decision-Making

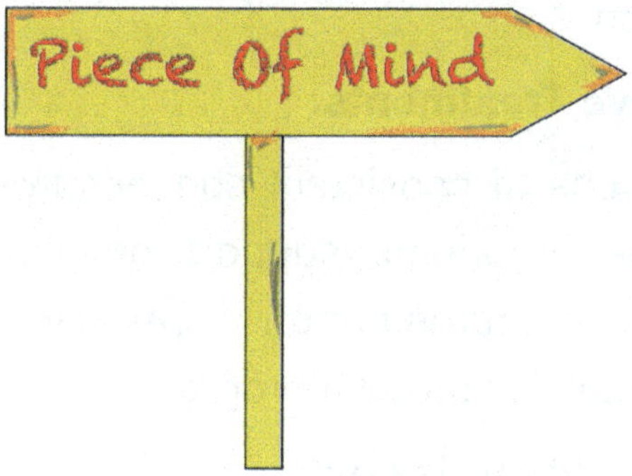

By seeking the opinion of a neurosurgeon specializing in craniocervical instability, a patient can confirm whether brain and spine conditions are contributing to their symptoms and better understand their surgical treatment option(s). Even if a patient's condition hasn't been definitively diagnosed by a neurosurgeon yet, knowing they've consulted a CCI neurosurgeon(s) can provide reassurance that they are on the right path toward addressing their health concerns. A focused evaluation can help patients feel more confident in their care decisions.

Even if a definitive diagnosis has not yet been made, assessing symptoms, obtaining the best imaging for ruling out CCI, being under the care of a conservative treatment healthcare team for at least 6 months, completing applicable quality of life and disability questionnaires, and consulting a CCI neurosurgeon(s) can provide valuable reassurance and guide patients through the process with confidence.

Chapter 1 Summary

Understanding when to consult a neurosurgeon is a key step in effectively managing craniocervical instability, especially when symptoms significantly impact daily life or conservative treatments have failed. Patients can initiate the proposed neurosurgical consultation decision-making framework process themselves, with a physician or better yet, a supportive and knowledgable healthcare team. However, patients experiencing severe symptoms should always seek urgent medical care.

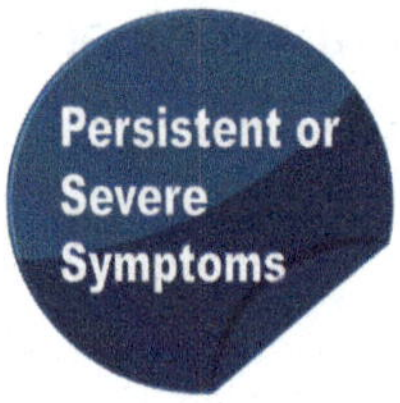

Decision Factor #1 – Severe or Frequent Symptoms:
Patients should track their most severe and frequent symptoms using rating tools like the Likert scale (impact), pain scale (0–10), and frequency scale. A one-page summary listing symptoms by severity, frequency, and onset date may help guide timely neurosurgical evaluation.

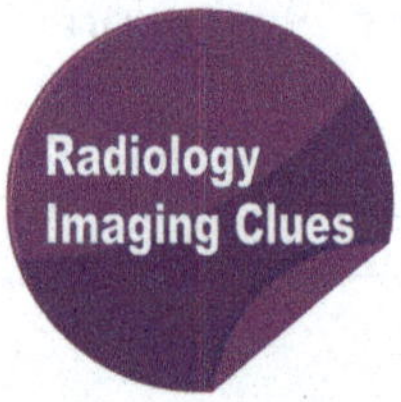

Decision Factor #2 – Imaging to Rule Out CCI & Comorbidities:

Basic imaging to evaluate CCI includes upright dynamic cervical 3D CT and MRI (or supine MRI Cervical Spine) and MRI Brain. These should assess for instability and related conditions. Radiology reports should be done by specialists experienced in CCI and if the reports indicate abnormalities, it may help guide timely neurosurgical evaluation.

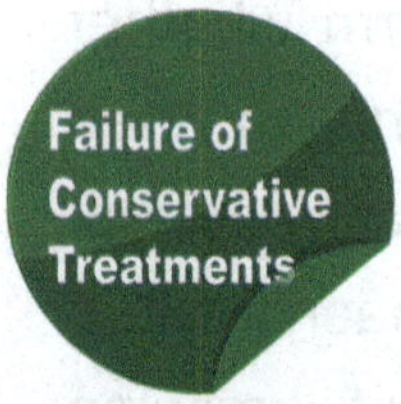

Decision Factor #3 – Failure of Conservative Treatments:

If symptoms persist or worsen after ~ 6 months of consistent conservative care, including physical therapy, medications, ergonomic support, bracing, and other treatments, patients should consult a neurosurgeon, especially if neurological symptoms or high mechanical irritability prevent progress.

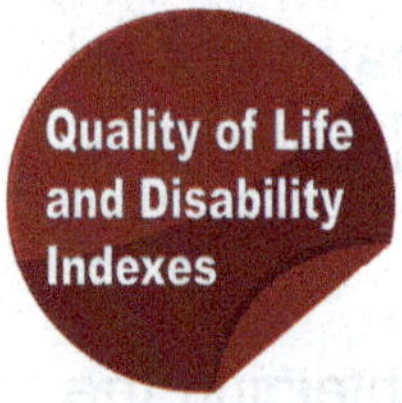

Decision Factor #4 – Quality of Life & Disability Indexes:

If chronic symptoms significantly reduce quality of life or daily functioning as shown by tools like the SF-36, NDI, EQ-5D, Karnofsky, or MoCA, it may be time to consult a neurosurgeon, especially when conservative care fails to restore independence or well-being.

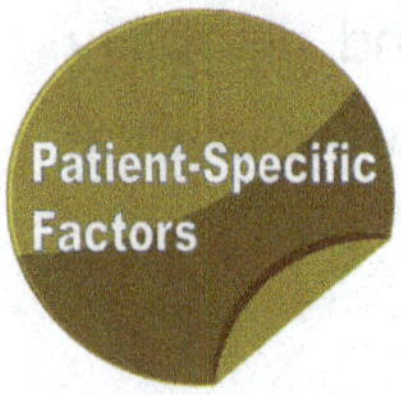

Decision Factor #5 – Patient-Specific Factors:

Age, overall health, comorbidities, and the need for diagnostic clarity all affect surgical decisions, and consulting a CCI-focused neurosurgeon can help weigh risks, confirm diagnosis, and provide peace of mind.

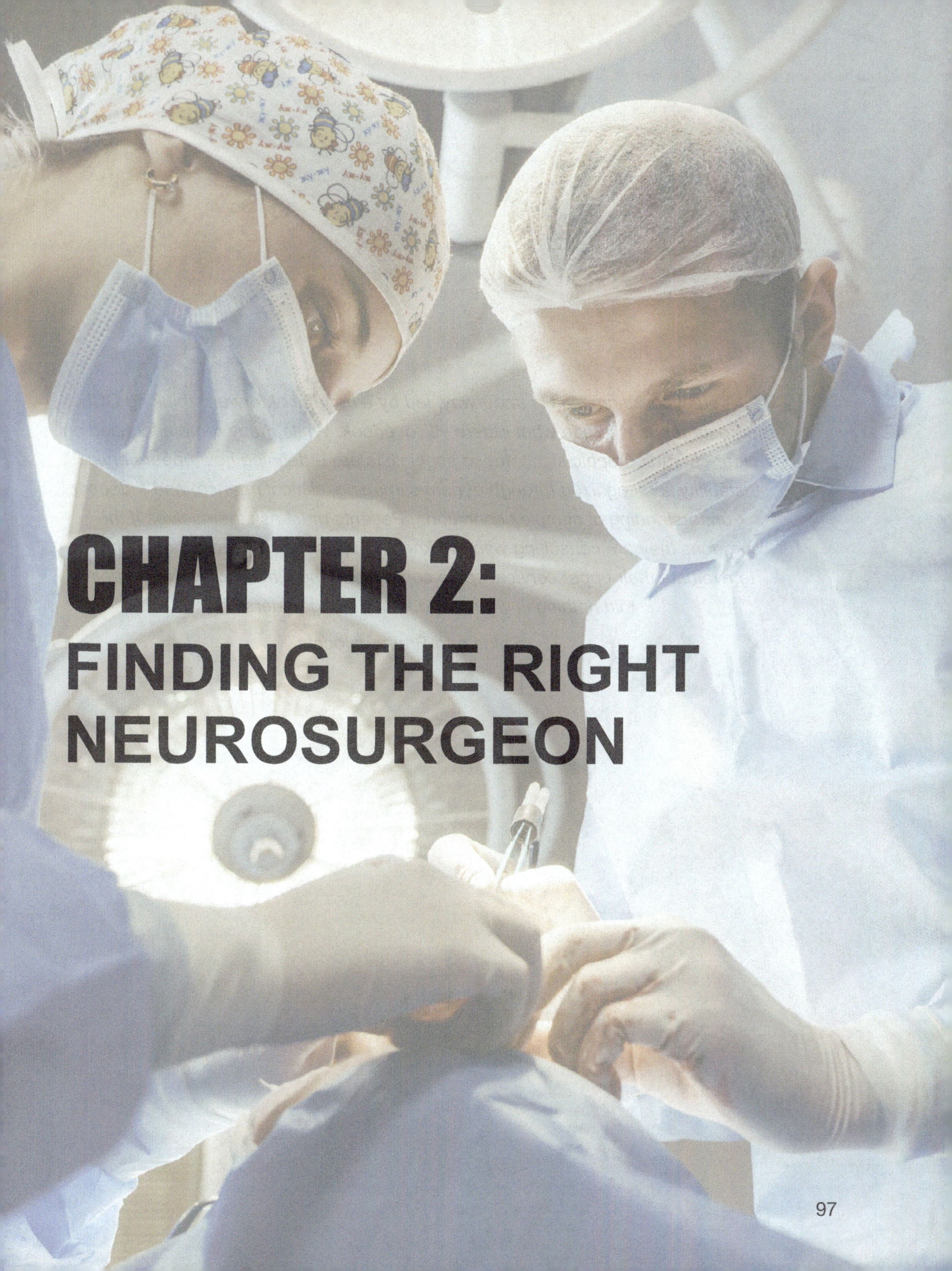

CHAPTER 2:

FINDING THE RIGHT NEUROSURGEON

"A quiet paradigm shift is underway, led by a handful of forward-thinking CCI neurosurgeons who see what others still overlook. While many remain focused on clear-cut radiographic signs, these specialists are redefining how upper cervical instability is recognized through dynamic imaging, clinical nuance, and a deeper understanding of complex conditions. Patients must ask themselves if the surgeons they are consulting with are keeping up, because who patients choose to evaluate their upper cervical spine could mean the difference between being told nothing is wrong and finally being understood."

- Spine and Brain Advocate

Introduction

Choosing the right neurosurgeon for craniocervical instability (CCI) is one of the most critical decisions a patient will make in their CCI healthcare journey. This condition is complex, under-diagnosed, and often misunderstood, making it essential to find specialists with the appropriate expertise and approach. Below is a general guide of what to look for and consider when selecting a neurosurgeon, but first, a practical surgical overview will help provide patients with a basic understanding of craniocervical fusion (CCF) surgeries before they start looking for a neurosurgeon.

When seeking a neurosurgeon or consulting with physicians in general, it's important to have patience and realistic expectations. Not all doctors will be familiar with, or up to date on, complex conditions like craniocervical instability (CCI) or related disorders. These are nuanced, evolving areas of medicine, and finding the right specialist may take time and persistence. Advocating for yourself or your loved one, while remaining respectful and informed, can make a significant difference in receiving appropriate care.

A Brief History of Craniocervical Fusion Surgery

Atlanto-Occipital and atlantoaxial fusion surgeries became mainstream medical practices in the latter half of the 20th century. These techniques were developed to treat severe instability of the upper cervical spine, particularly at the junction between the skull and the second cervical vertebra, which is called Atlanto-occipital fusion (OCF), and between C1 and C2, which is called Atlantoaxial fusion (AAF). The first documented attempts to fuse these areas surgically began in the 1950s, with significant advancements in the 1970s and 1990s. The development of better surgical instruments, the mainstream use of CT imaging in the early to mid 1980s, and a greater understanding of spine biomechanics allowed these surgeries to become more reliable and effective.

These fusion procedures were first used to treat internal decapitation, a serious injury that can result from severe trauma, Down syndrome, a bone problem called os odontoideum, rheumatoid arthritis, Grisel's syndrome (a rare condition that can happen after an upper respiratory infection in children), and tumors in the upper part of the neck. In the past, physicians only suspected upper cervical instability in these specific types of cases. Other conditions or injuries were rarely considered likely to cause instability at the craniocervical junction.

These fusion procedures were especially important for treating very evident cases where the bones in the craniocervical area were obviously out of place. This misalignment could usually be seen during a physical exam or on basic MRI or CT scans taken while the patient was lying down. This problem could cause pressure on the spinal cord and brainstem, and surgery was only done in cases that were life-threatening.

By the early 2000s, techniques such as the Goel-Harms method, along with the use of improved spinal hardware, had further refined upper cervical fusion surgeries, establishing them as the gold standard for stabilizing the upper cervical spine. Over time, improvements in surgical methods and instrumentation have led to higher success rates, making these procedures vital for restoring craniocervical stability and preventing neurological complications.

In the last decade or so, a growing number of leading neurosurgeons recognize that the craniocervical junction can be affected not only by the traditional factors listed above, but also in chronic inflammatory conditions, chronic infections, patients with connective tissue disorders such as Ehlers-Danlos Syndrome, and trauma cases where the instability was overlooked. This increased attention was due in part to advancements in imaging techniques such as upright and dynamic positions of head and neck flexion, extension and rotation, and a better understanding of the condition's impact on neurological function.

As a result, there is a specialized group of neurosurgeons who are knowledgeable in diagnosing and treating CCI, including occult cases of CCI and AAI. Within this group, an even smaller subset of neurosurgeons focuses specifically on CCI in the context of EDS, Complex Chiari, and commonly associated comorbidities.

These highly specialized CCI neurosurgeons take a holistic and advanced approach to diagnosis and treatment. They do not rely solely on measurements or static imaging; instead, dynamic imaging plays a crucial role in their assessments.

With the skill to accurately interpret complex imaging alongside a comprehensive evaluation of symptoms, and tests, they grasp the complexity of this injury. Their expertise extends beyond traditional causes as they recognize connections to chronic infections involving conditions such as mast cells, hypermobility and connective tissue disorders. Moreover, their advanced approach has enabled them to identify “occult” cases of instability caused by trauma. For example, one study indicated 6.45% of traumatic occult (hidden / not visible) AOD cases were missed by neurosurgeons who relied on the traditional standard, supine medical imaging measurements and obvious neurological signs (unconscious, gait issues etc.)

In recent years, emerging research suggests potential common CCI comorbidities including hypermobility, EDS, Eagle syndrome, mast cell activation syndrome (MCAS), and adult tethered cord, to name a few. These other conditions could explain the patient's symptoms and should be evaluated or ruled out before arriving at a final diagnosis(es). Dedicated research teams are actively working to better understand these complex conditions and develop more effective non-invasive tests and successful treatments.

These developments represent a major step forward in surgical care. For patients with complex conditions and multiple diagnoses, finding a neurosurgeon who not only specializes in CCI but also stays up to date with the latest research can be an important step toward getting the most informed and effective care.

Atlanto-occipital and atlantoaxial fusion procedures, now also termed craniocervical fusion, are cornerstone techniques in spinal stabilization for patients with traumatic injuries, congenital anomalies, inflammatory conditions, or degenerative changes that have led to instability of the upper cervical spine. While several approaches have been refined over time, the success of these procedures ultimately depends on the surgeon's experience, anatomical familiarity, and adaptability to each patient's unique pathology as well as the patient's overall health.

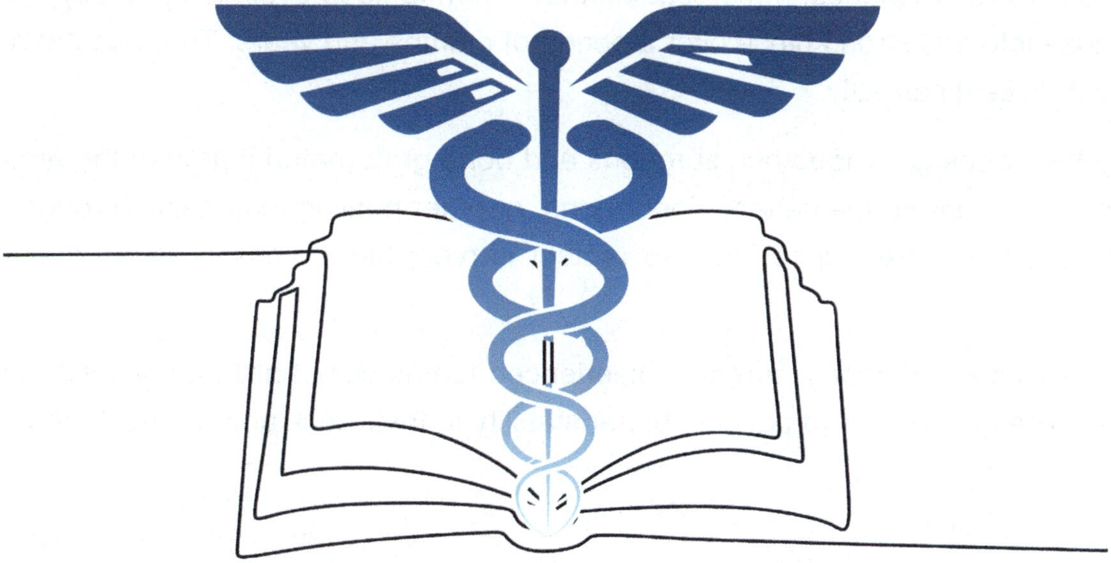

Overview of Craniocervical Fusion Surgery

Craniocervical fusion (CCF) is a surgery that helps stabilize the area where the skull meets the top of the neck. This surgery includes:

- Occipito-cervical fusion (OCF), which joins the base of the skull (occiput) to the second neck bone (C2), also termed Atlanto-occipital fusion (AOF); or
- Atlantoaxial fusion (AAF), which joins the first neck bone (C1) to the second neck bone (C2)

These procedures are used to treat instability or "looseness" in these respective parts of the spine. CCF surgery is only done after a thorough assessment. It aims to stop or reduce pressure on the nerves, blood vessels, spinal cord and brainstem caused by unstable bones. Over time, surgeons have improved the procedure to make it safer and more effective, especially for people with smaller bones or conditions like EDS.

During surgery, the surgeon places small screws into the skull and neck bones. The exact position depends on the patient's unique anatomy to avoid harming nearby important parts like nerves, blood vessels, muscles, and the spinal cord. Sometimes, small veins are tied off, and the joints between the skull and neck bones are gently opened to help the bones heal together.

Surgeons use special tools and live imaging to carefully insert screws at the right angle. After the screws are placed, metal rods connect them to keep everything steady while the bones fuse into one strong piece over a period of months and years. The rods are shaped to fit each patient perfectly.

To help the bones grow together, surgeons add bone graft material around the area. This can include bone from the patient, donor bone, or other healing materials. Throughout the surgery, the team takes great care to protect nerves, blood vessels, and other critical parts.

Even though it is a complex surgery, experienced teams work hard to make it as safe as possible. The goal is to give patients better stability in their neck and protect their nervous system.

Caregiver Support Matters When Finding a Neurosurgeon

Searching for the right neurosurgeon(s) to consult with can be overwhelming. The process involves more than just booking an appointment. Patients often need to research multiple specialists, understand different treatment philosophies, gather medical records and imaging, fill out detailed intake forms and correspond with healthcare teams through emails and sometimes advanced technology. Each neurosurgeon or clinic may have their own unique process, requirements, and expectations, which adds to the confusion and workload.

This journey can be both mentally and emotionally exhausting. Patients are already dealing with pain, fatigue, or neurological symptoms that affect their ability to think clearly or stay organized. On top of that, there can be anxiety and fear about the future, the diagnosis, or whether surgery might be necessary. Trying to manage all of this alone can feel like a full-time job, and for some, it becomes just that.

Having caregiver support during this process can make a big difference. Primary care doctors, physiotherapists, upper cervical chiropractors, Health Psychologist or Clinical Health Psychologist, or other healthcare providers can help identify which specialists to consider and may provide referrals or letters of medical necessity. Paid patient advocates or asking a family member or friend to be a temporary care coordinator to assist with collecting medical records, organizing imaging, or even writing out symptom histories and timelines can be extremely helpful. Even trusted friends, a partner, or community volunteers can help make a few phone calls, track communication, or attend appointments.

While many patients do handle this process alone, having a support system can reduce stress and help ensure that nothing gets missed. It can also help patients pace themselves and feel less overwhelmed.

Remember, patients asking for help is not a sign of weakness, it's a smart way to stay focused on their health and make informed decisions. Seeking multiple opinions is often necessary, and having support can help patients navigate the system and find the neurosurgeon that is the right fit for their needs and values.

10 Key Things To Look For When Selecting A Neurosurgeon

1. Specializes in Conditions of the Craniocervical Junction

Finding a neurosurgeon who specializes in conditions related to the craniocervical junction (CCJ) is critical. Unlike brain or spine neurosurgical issues, conditions of the craniocervical junction require a highly specialized and multifaceted approach due to its unique and complex anatomy and proximity to the brainstem, cranial nerves, vertebral arteries, and respiratory centers, and one that not all neurosurgeons have experiences.

Many neurosurgeons have a “niche expertise” or what the medical field calls a “subspecialty”. For example, some neurosurgeons specialize in neurovascular nerve-related compression syndromes such as Helps or Vancouver syndromes, which happens when blood vessels compress specific cranial nerves. Other neurosurgery subspecialties include cranial/brain neurosurgery, spine neurosurgeons, functional neurosurgery, vascular neurosurgery, trauma neurosurgery, neuro-oncology, and endovascular neurosurgery.

When searching for a neurosurgeon, it is essential for patients to find one with specific expertise in diagnosing and treating CCI. These specialists are highly skilled at identifying subtle signs of CCI and have developed a comprehensive, detailed approach to ruling out CCI. Their specialized training and clinical experience enable them to detect abnormalities at the craniocervical junction that may be missed by other neurosurgeons. Ultimately, selecting a neurosurgeon with a specialization in CCI can significantly impact a patient’s ability to receive an accurate diagnosis and effective treatment.

Many neurosurgeons focus on treating patients whose lives are seriously affected by conditions involving the craniocervical junction. Patients are generally considered for surgery if their symptoms significantly reduce their quality of life, such as being unable to work full-time, patients with large syringomyelia cavities (a fluid-filled cyst within the spinal cord), serious neurological symptoms, or severe abnormalities seen on imaging because these cases are more likely to worsen over time. Each neurosurgeon follows their own patient selection criteria to ensure that patients with the most urgent medical needs receive timely care. This highlights that even if patients find a neurosurgeon who specializes in the craniocervical junction or CCI, many of these neurosurgeons focus on patients whose symptoms are severe and significantly impact their daily lives, such as those unable to work full-time or who have progressive neurological issues.

2. Understands the Complexity of a CCI Diagnosis

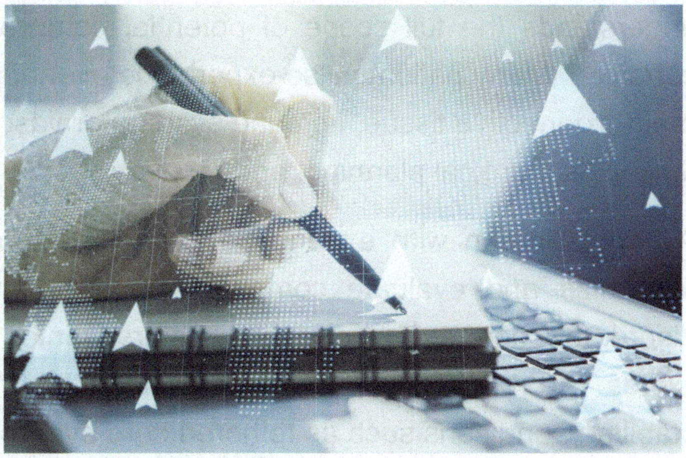

CCI can cause a wide range of symptoms, including neck pain, dizziness, cognitive issues, and neurological changes. These symptoms often mimic other conditions, which makes diagnosing CCI especially difficult. That's why it's important for patients to find a neurosurgeon who specializes in the craniocervical junction and understands the complex nature of CCI.

A neurosurgeon with experience in CCI goes beyond standard evaluations. They take into account the full spectrum of symptoms, including how much the condition affects daily activities, mobility, and overall well-being. Rather than focusing only on severe signs like paralysis or walking difficulties, they evaluate how the condition impacts a patient's ability to function and enjoy life. Their goal is to carefully assess a lot of information to either confirm or rule out a CCI diagnosis.

These specialists also recognize that CCI is not always visible on regular imaging tests like static MRIs or CT scans. For this reason, they often rely on dynamic imaging such as scans taken such as upright or flexion-extension-rotation MRIs, which capture spinal alignment in various positions. Just as important, they know how to interpret these test results in the context of the patient's full clinical picture.

For patients who may have CCI, it is essential to find a neurosurgeon who has the right knowledge, experience, and diagnostic tools. Choosing a CCI neurosurgeon who truly understands the complexity of CCI can lead to a more accurate diagnosis and better treatment options.

3. Knowledge of Common CCI-Related Comorbidities

When seeking care for CCI, it is essential that patients find a neurosurgeon who understands the full scope of potential comorbid conditions. CCI is rarely an isolated condition. Many patients also experience overlapping conditions that may affect the spine, brain, connective tissue, immune system, or vascular system, each of which can influence diagnosis, surgical planning, and recovery.

A neurosurgeon with experience in these interconnected issues is better equipped to recognize and evaluate complex symptom patterns. For example, connective tissue disorders such as hypermobile Ehlers-Danlos Syndrome (hEDS) or immune-related issues like Mast Cell Activation Syndrome (MCAS) can affect surgical healing and stability. Conditions such as tethered cord syndrome and Eagle syndrome may need to be addressed first to ensure a safer and more effective surgical outcome.

Many of these comorbidities are subtle, under-diagnosed, or require multidisciplinary care. A neurosurgeon who routinely screens patients, or refers them to specialists as necessary, is more likely to develop a treatment plan that is both safer and more personalized. This means developing a plan that accounts for the full range of contributing factors rather than solely focusing on CCI.

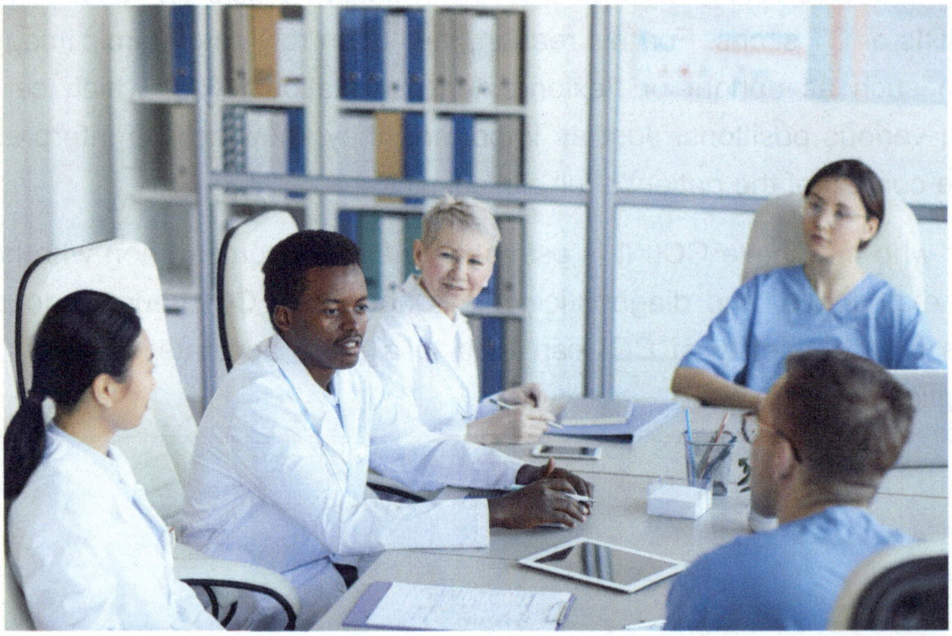

Not all neurosurgeons are trained to identify or manage these associated conditions. If overlooked, these comorbidities may result in incomplete care or suboptimal outcomes.

For this reason, it is crucial that each patient selects a specialist who supports them in taking a comprehensive approach. Patients with Ehlers-Danlos Syndrome (EDS), in particular, should always consult with surgeons who have specific expertise in managing EDS-related complexities.

A thorough understanding of these factors is key to building a safe, effective, and individualized treatment plan. Here is a list of some possible comorbid conditions:

- Eagle syndrome (jugular, nerve)
- Cranial Nerve Compression
- Intracranial Pressure (ICP) or Cerebral Venous Congestion
- Vertebral Artery Compression or Kinking
- Sub-axial cervical spine instability or abnormalities (C3-T1)
- Adult Occult Tethered Cord
- Chiari Malformation
- Basilar Invagination
- Loss of cervical lordosis or kyphosis

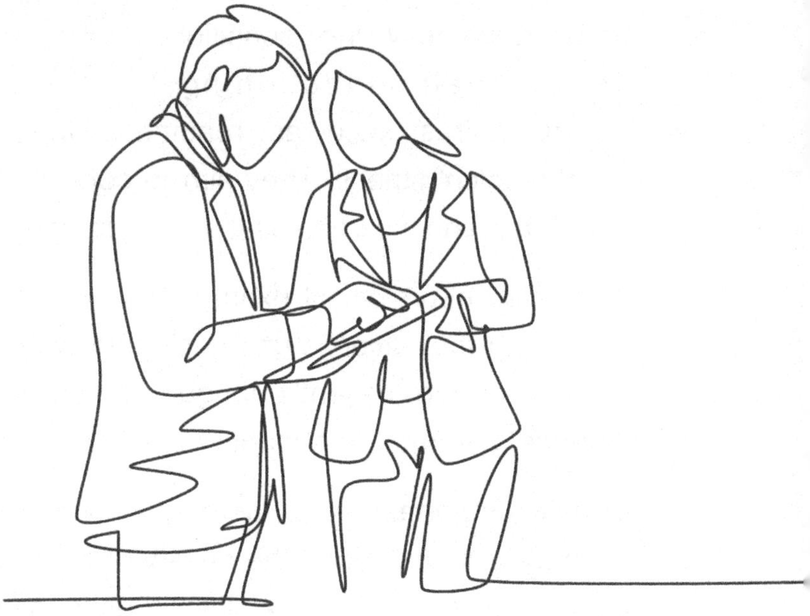

4. Completes A Comprehensive Assessment of Each Patient

When choosing a neurosurgeon, it's important to find a specialist who performs a thorough and structured assessment before recommending procedures like craniocervical fusion. This process should be formal, comprehensive, and guided by clear clinical reasoning. Surgery should only be considered after carefully evaluating whether it is truly necessary and appropriate for the patient.

A qualified CCI neurosurgeon begins with a detailed medical history and a series of diagnostic evaluations. These may include genetic testing such as Ehlers-Danlos syndrome (EDS) panels, particularly for vascular EDS, screening for Marfan syndrome and other connective tissue disorders, pharmacogenetic testing, comprehensive blood work (including thyroid function, vitamin D, calcium, prolactin, adrenal, and others, like hormonal markers), a 24-hour cortisol test, metal allergy testing, and thorough physical and neurological examinations.

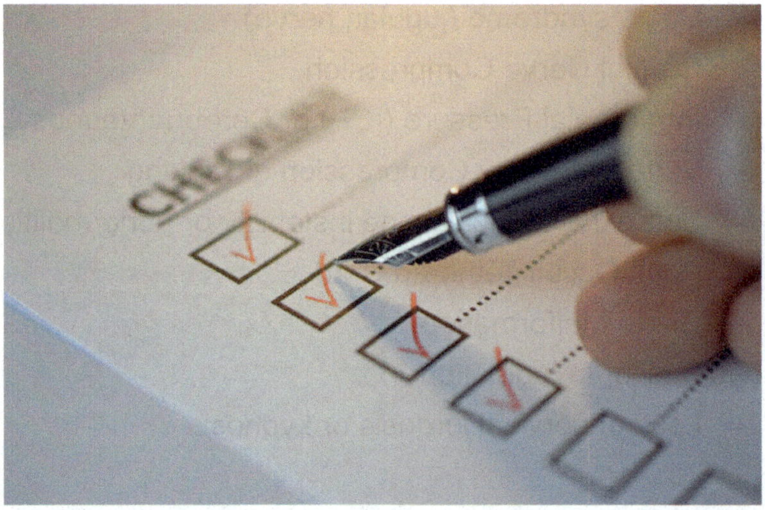

They often use symptom checklists, disability scales, quality-of-life assessments to understand how the condition affects daily functioning, questionnaires such as readiness for surgery, bone frailty, mental fatigue, and psychological fitness. They aim to confirm the diagnosis, rule out other possible causes, and determine if surgery is the best course of action.

A detailed neurological exam is a key part of this process. This includes things such as assessing the patient's gait (including walking on toes and heels), neurological exam by looking at the patient's tongue, finger test (Hoffman's sign), reflexes, coordination, balance, and muscle strength to identify signs of brainstem or spinal cord involvement.

Equally important is a thorough review of the patient's symptoms, their frequency, severity, and impact on the quality of their daily life. Patients are often asked to complete quality of life and disability questionnaires, which help the neurosurgeon better understand how the condition is affecting their patient's overall function and well-being.

The neurosurgeon will also review any non-surgical treatments already attempted by the patient, such as physical therapy, medications, or bracing, and will evaluate how effective those approaches have been. Additional tests and advanced imaging are often required to provide a complete understanding of the condition.

Lastly, a CCI neurosurgeon understands that comorbidities are often present in patients with CCI and will conduct a thorough differential diagnosis. They may collaborate with other specialists to help rule out or confirm these comorbidities and, ideally, work together to determine the most appropriate treatment plan for each patient's unique case.

This comprehensive, patient-centered approach ensures surgery is only recommended when fully supported by clinical, functional, and radiological evidence, leading to more accurate diagnoses, better outcomes, and fewer unnecessary procedures.

5. Recognizes Subtle Abnormalities in Radiology Images

It is important for patients to choose a neurosurgeon who is skilled in identifying subtle abnormalities or occult CCI through radiology images. Many general radiologists and neurosurgeons focus only on clear issues, such as spinal cord compression or traumatic fractures, often relying on static, supine imaging like standard MRIs or CT scans. However, conditions affecting the CCJ often involve small or hidden signs on static imaging, or may only appear when the head or neck is in certain positions.

A neurosurgeon with true expertise in CCI knows how to detect subtle signs of craniocervical instability. They use advanced, dynamic imaging techniques, including flexion, extension, and rotational views. They also rely on multiple types of imaging such as MRI, CT scans, angiograms, venograms, and even motion X-ray videos to get a full and accurate view of the patient's anatomy in movement.

High-quality imaging is essential for making the right diagnosis. Upright and dynamic MRI and CT scans of the cervical spine are especially helpful for detecting instability that may not be visible on standard, lying-down (supine) scans. Brain MRIs are also important for checking related conditions like Chiari malformation, cerebrospinal fluid (CSF) leaks, venous congestion, or intracranial hypertension. Thin-slice 1 mm dynamic CT scans offer detailed views of bone structures and are especially useful for accurate CCJ measurements, ruling out elongated or abnormal styloid processes (structures in the neck) and surgical planning.

Specialists experienced in CCI use a range of important measurements such as the clivo-axial angle, Grabb-Oakes line, and Harris measurements, not only in a neutral position but also while the head and neck are in different positions.

Some patients may appear stable in a neutral position but show clear signs of instability during flexion, extension and rotation. These neurosurgeons also recognize the value of upright imaging, which factor in the force of gravity and can reveal problems missed by standard lying down scans.

In addition to using key measurements, experienced neurosurgeons look for other subtle signs on imaging. These include degeneration or damage in the joints between C1, C2, condyles, and the base of the skull, osteoarthritis, facet and ligament injuries, and abnormal compression or twisting of blood vessels, Tarlov cysts, sinus dehiscence, C1/ styloid process abnormalities, and calcification or elongation of the stylohyoid ligament. They may also detect issues with the optic nerve, spinal discs, empty sella, and other signs of intracranial hypertension.

Traditionally, Chiari I Malformation has been diagnosed when the cerebellar tonsils extend 5 mm or more below the foramen magnum. However, experts now recognize that this 5 mm cutoff is somewhat arbitrary and does not consider other important anatomical factors. Some patients with less than 5 mm of tonsillar descent can still have significant symptoms and may benefit from surgery. A skilled neurosurgeon evaluates the entire structure of the brain and spine, including CSF flow and positional dynamics, rather than relying on a single measurement.

By choosing a neurosurgeon with this level of knowledge and experience, patients can be confident that even the most subtle signs of CCI will be identified, leading to more accurate diagnoses and personalized treatment plans.

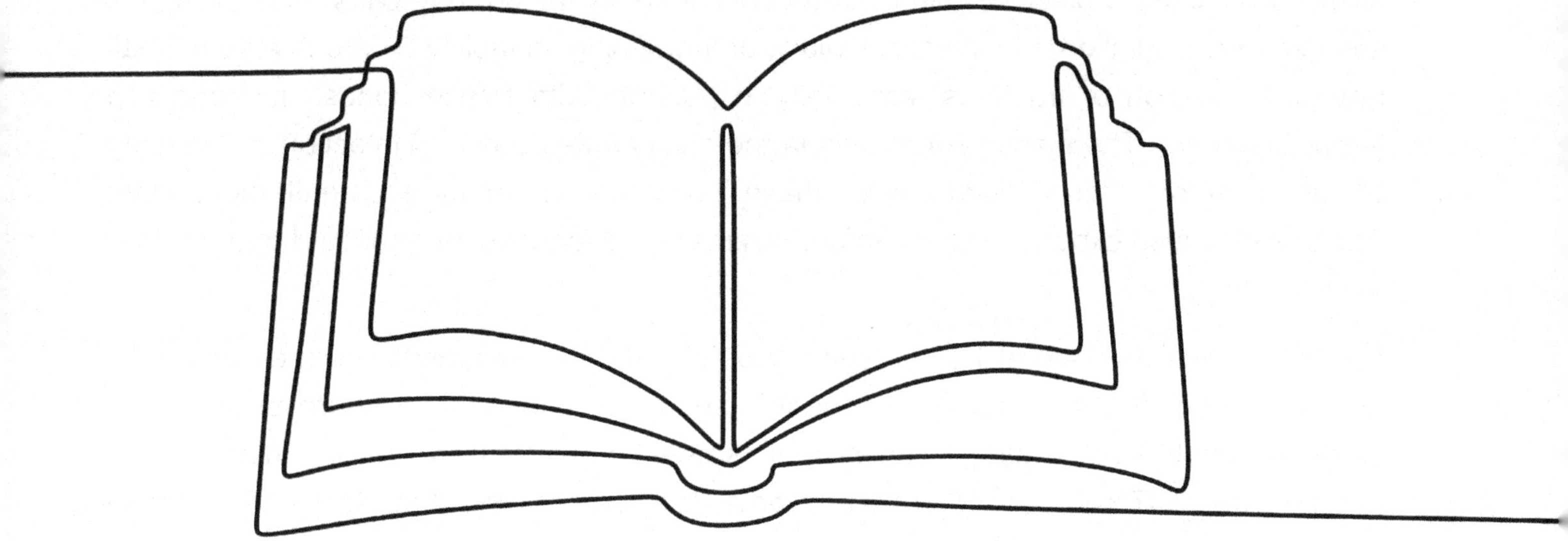

6. Expertise in The Role of Invasive Cervical Traction

The process of cervical traction often begins with manual traction, where gentle pulling of the head and neck is done by hand to determine if symptoms improve. Even when traditional scans appear normal or show only borderline abnormalities, a positive response to manual traction can point toward an underlying vertical instability in the upper spine.

If manual traction brings symptom relief, the next step may be invasive cervical traction (ICT). This involves attaching a traction device to the skull using small pins and gradually applying controlled pulling force on the neck while taking real-time X-rays (fluoroscopy). These images allow the surgeon to observe how the skull and upper spine move and align during traction. ICT helps confirm the diagnosis in certain cases of CCI but also simulates the potential results of surgery, guiding the surgeon in planning the most effective approach. Intracranial pressure (ICP) bolt monitoring may also be used to assess brain pressure changes.

In cases of suspected vertical instability, where the skull may be sliding down over the spine, ICT is *specifically* useful. However, ICT is an invasive procedure and does carry risks for patients. It places strain on the cervical spine, which may cause complications such as nerve irritation, blood vessel injury, or worsening instability. There is also a small risk of dislocation or fractures, especially in patients with fragile bones or connective tissue disorders. The placement of pins in the skull carries a risk of infection or bleeding at the insertion sites. Though rare, these complications require careful monitoring. Patients may also experience discomfort, dizziness, headaches, or nausea during or after the procedure.

Due to its invasive nature, ICT is typically used only after less invasive methods have been explored. It should always be performed by an experienced neurosurgeon in a carefully controlled setting with proper safety measures in place. When used appropriately, ICT can provide critical insights into some cases of vertical CCI and help guide safer, more personalized treatment plans.

7. Extensive Surgical Experience and Use of Precision Alignment Technology

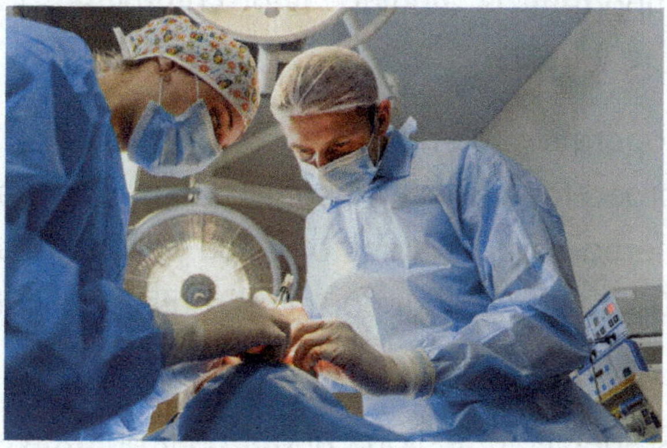

When considering a neurosurgical consultation for ruling out or confirming CCI, it is essential for patients to select a neurosurgeon who has extensive fusion surgery experience and uses advanced technology to ensure proper alignment before performing the fusion. These surgeries involve the most sensitive and important part of the spine, where the surgeon must be very careful to protect the nerves, blood vessels, and spinal cord and keep the head and neck properly aligned and stable over time.

Leading neurosurgeons in this subspecialty often have decades of focused experience and have performed thousands of craniocervical fusion (CCF) and atlantoaxial fusion (AAF) surgeries, some experts performing 1,000 to over 4,000 surgical cases. High surgical volume is a strong indicator of expertise and is associated with better outcomes and fewer complications.

Due to the anatomical complexity and individual variability of each case, a personalized surgical approach is key. Patients requiring occiput-to-C2 (Oc–C2) fusion benefit from selecting a surgeon with a proven track record in craniocervical fusion. Likewise, those with atlantoaxial instability should seek a surgeon skilled in procedures such as the Goel-Harms technique, widely regarded as the gold standard for atlantoaxial fusion.

In this highly specialized area of neurosurgery, general experience with spinal procedures may not be sufficient. Optimal results are achieved by neurosurgeons who routinely perform the exact operation required, who possess a deep understanding of the condition being treated and who utilize intraoperative navigation (i.e., a tool that helps surgeons see exactly where they are operating inside the body in real time, using images from scans like CT or MRI) and imaging technologies to ensure precise anatomical alignment prior to fixation and fusion. For rare and complex spinal pathologies, surgical expertise must match the complexity of the diagnosis. Choosing a surgeon who specializes in the precise fusion procedure needed is one of the most important steps toward achieving surgical safety, spinal stability, and long-term success.

8. Committed to Follow-Up Care

When undergoing fusion surgery for CCI choosing a neurosurgeon with diagnostic and surgical expertise is essential, but equally important is finding one committed to comprehensive follow-up care.

Unfortunately, some patients report poor postoperative communication and support, especially those who travel from out of town or abroad for surgery. In some cases, serious concerns such as new symptoms, suspected tethered cord, or signs of failed fusion have gone unanswered for long periods of time. This lack of support can delay critical interventions and compromise recovery.

Before committing to surgery, patients should ask specific questions about post-operative care policies. Will the surgeon provide ongoing follow-up through tele-health or in-person visits? Will the surgeon order follow up imaging to assess fusion progress? Do they collaborate or refer patients to CCF-knowledgeable occupational therapists, physiotherapists and other specialists? How do they respond to complications, and will they coordinate care with a patient's local healthcare providers?

According to the American College of Surgeons' Statement on Principles, *surgeons are responsible not only for the surgery itself but also for pre-operative planning and post-operative monitoring.* However, this statement does not indicate the specifics of the duration of post-operative monitoring. This includes managing complications and ensuring continuity of care. If a surgeon's practice does not reflect this standard, it is important to clarify in advance what support can be realistically expected.

A knowledgeable and dedicated neurosurgeon specializing in CCF will not only perform the procedure but also help guide recovery, and ensure that complications and concerns are addressed, and work with the patient's broader care team, including a CCF knowledge physiotherapist. In short, a neurosurgeon should remain a patient's partner in care, not just during surgery, but up to 1 year or more post-surgery.

9. Location and Travel Logistics

For many patients seeking treatment for CCI and CCF, finding a skilled neurosurgeon may mean traveling long distances, sometimes even out of the country. While this can be a significant challenge, ensuring that patients receive specialized care for such a complex condition is essential.

Given that CCI is a rare and complex condition, it's likely that local options may not have the necessary expertise. In many cases, patients must travel to centers of specialized neurosurgeons or clinics that have experience in diagnosing and treating CCI. Traveling for treatment is often the only way to access the advanced care and surgical skill required to properly address CCI and related complications.

When considering an out-of-town or out-of-country surgeon, it's important to understand the logistics of the process. Travel time and recovery requirements will need to be factored in. Most patients must stay near the hospital for several weeks following surgery to ensure proper recovery before receiving a fit-to-travel or fit-to-fly certificate. During this period, patients must ensure that post-operative care and recovery support are available locally or that the hospital has a recovery plan in place.

One of the biggest challenges when traveling abroad for surgery is ensuring patients have adequate post-surgery support. Since follow-up care will likely be limited, it's crucial to research whether the patient's home country's healthcare system can provide assistance after they return home. This includes confirming that local doctors or healthcare providers are willing to assist with complications or follow-up procedures, should they arise. Another critical factor is ensuring insurance covers care abroad, including surgery, post-op care, and potential complications. If surgery is out of network or patients do not have health insurance, they will need to explore what out-of-pocket costs may arise.

Although traveling for surgery can be difficult, it's crucial that patients with complex conditions like CCI receive care from a neurosurgeon who can meet their needs and limitations. When choosing a surgeon, patients may want to consider how close the specialist is to their home, as proximity can help with follow-up care and recovery.

10. Personal and Communicative Fit

For patients facing the complex condition of CCI, it's important to look for a surgeon who is not only highly skilled, but also approachable and communicative. Finding a neurosurgeon who is the “right fit” for individual patients can make a significant difference in how smooth and manageable the diagnosis and treatment process feels for the patient.

Patients can start by asking for referrals. Speaking with other patients who have faced similar challenges, or trusted healthcare providers who can offer helpful insight into a surgeon’s experience, communication style, and overall approach. Firsthand recommendations often reveal details that may not be found online.

A neurosurgeon’s communication style plays a big role as well. Patients benefit most from someone who can clearly explain complex medical issues, listens carefully, and welcomes questions. It’s equally important that caregivers, who often assist with appointments, medication management, and recovery, feel involved and supported by the neurosurgeon and staff throughout the process. The responsiveness of the surgeon’s office is another key factor. Understanding how communication is handled before and after surgery is helpful. For example, knowing who to contact with questions and the team’s response time policy can reduce unnecessary stress. Ultimately, the best fit is a surgeon who combines technical expertise with clear communication, values patient and caregiver input, and fosters a supportive, collaborative environment throughout the process.

In summary, choosing the right neurosurgeon who provides individualized care for CCI is critical. Looking for a specialist who not only understands the craniocervical junction, but also offers a comprehensive, patient-centered approach, is important. The best outcomes come from those who demonstrate subspecialty expertise, recognize subtle imaging abnormalities, assess comorbidities, and offer personalized diagnostics, surgical skill, and long-term support.

Summary of Things To Look For When Selecting A Neurosurgeon

- Specialization in the craniocervical junction and CCI
- Deep understanding of CCI complexity
- Familiarity with common comorbidities
- Comprehensive patient assessment
- Ability to detect subtle radiologic signs
- Skilled use of invasive cervical traction (if needed)
- High-volume surgical experience
- Strong commitment to follow-up care
- Support for travel and logistics
- Personal and communicative fit for the patient

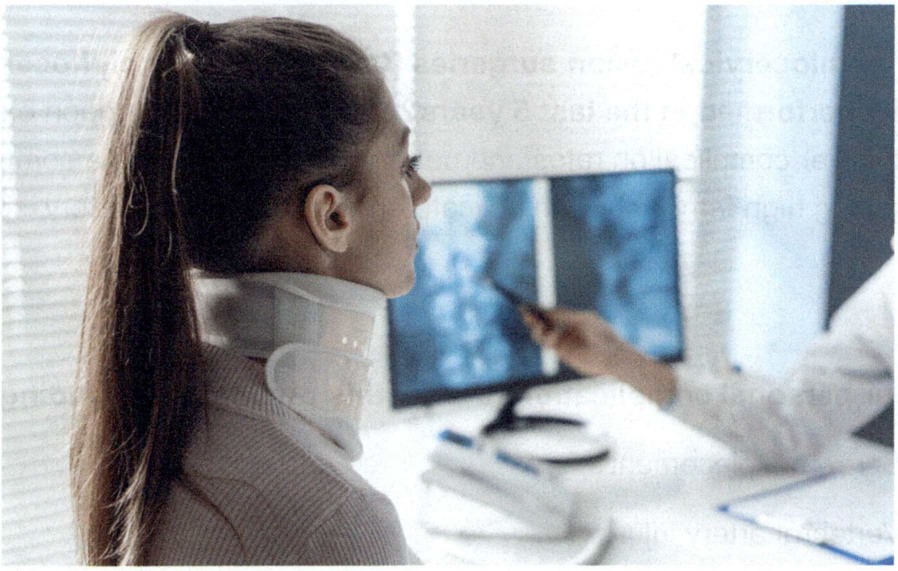

🔍 Sample Questions to Ask a Neurosurgeon Before Accepting CCF Surgery

Respectful Questions, Safer Outcomes

It's completely appropriate to ask neurosurgeon's questions in the consultation appointment. Providing questions in advance of the meeting can help neurosurgeons prepare for questions. Most skilled, ethical neurosurgeons welcome informed patients who ask thoughtful, relevant questions, with the goal of understanding risks and staying safe. Asking good questions shows that patients are advocating for your health, aware of the risks, likely to follow pre- and post-op care which improves recover outcomes. If a surgeon gets annoyed, dismissive, vague, or impatient when you ask about alignment, safety, or screw placement, it could be a sign of communication issues. Keeping tone respectful and curious and not challenging them, show that patients care. Bottom line, asking questions is responsible, and a great surgeon will respect patients more, not less, and their answers can be part of the determining if there is a good fit.

Sample Questions:

1. How many craniocervical fusion surgeries (C1–C2 and/or occipitocervical) have you personally performed in the last 5 years? Why it matters: Surgeon experience correlates with lower complication rates and better outcomes. CCF is a complex procedure requiring high familiarity with delicate anatomy (vertebral artery, spinal cord, etc.).

2. What is your personal complication rate for this procedure, including:

- Screw misplacement?
- Vertebral artery injury?
- Revision surgery?
- Nonunion (failed fusion)?
- Nerve injury?

Why it matters (Top 2 risks):

- Screw misplacement (24.5%) can cause nerve damage, misalignment, hardware failure, and need for revision.
- Blood vessel injury (1.2%–8.2%) can lead to stroke, bleeding, or death, particularly with C1–C2 screws.

3. Do you routinely use intraoperative navigation (e.g., CT-guided or 3D navigation) and real-time imaging (fluoroscopy) during screw placement? Why it matters: Improves accuracy of hardware placement and reduces risk of vertebral artery injury, screw misplacement, and dural tears.

4. Do you use neuro-monitoring during surgery? Why it matters: Monitors spinal cord and nerve function in real time to prevent neurological injury.

5. How do you assess and achieve proper spinal alignment during surgery? Why it matters: Misalignment can cause residual brainstem compression, poor outcomes, or revision surgery. Some surgeons still rely mostly on their "feel" instead of measurable imaging alignment.

6. Do you use preoperative traction? If so, how is alignment confirmed before fixation? Why it matters: Proper traction and reduction of instability before fusion can improve long-term alignment and neurological outcomes.

7. What hardware system do you prefer for this procedure and why?

Ask specifically about:

- Use of occipital condyle screws (OCS) vs. traditional occipital plates
- Use of transarticular screws vs. C1 lateral mass and C2 pedicle screws

Why it matters: Low-profile hardware (e.g., occipital condyle screws) may reduce complications like hardware prominence and wound problems. Proper choice reduces revision risk.

8. What is your revision rate, and what are the most common reasons for re-operation in your patients? Why it matters: High revision rates can reflect problems with surgical technique, poor fusion rates, or hardware failure.

9. How do you assess for bone quality pre-surgery and optimize bone healing? Why it matters: Osteopenia and osteoporosis increase the risk of hardware failure and nonunion. Patients with EDS or chronic inflammatory conditions may have weaker bones.

10. How long do you expect bone fusion to take in my case, and how will fusion progress be monitored? Why it matters: Fusion can take 6–12 months or longer. Incomplete fusion increases hardware stress and risk of failure (e.g., screw breakage, loosening).

11. What is your post-operative care plan, including bracing, activity restrictions, and follow-up imaging? Why it matters: Clear post-op care reduces complications and promotes successful fusion. A rigid collar or halo vest may be needed in some cases.

12. How do you minimize infection risk, and what is your wound infection rate? Why it matters: Even low infection rates (0.5%–7.7%) can lead to major issues, including additional surgery.

13. How do you screen for or manage vertebral artery anomalies pre-surgery? Why it matters: High-riding vertebral arteries increase risk of artery injury during screw placement, especially at C2. 3D or 4D CTA or MRA should be done.

14. Have you treated patients with my specific medical condition(s) (EDS, osteopenia, trauma, etc.)? Why it matters: Some causes of CCI (e.g., Ehlers-Danlos Syndrome) involve tissue fragility, comorbidities, and need special care. Experience in your diagnosis is critical.

15. Do you use advanced imaging pre-operation? Why it matters: Advanced preoperative imaging (CT, MRI, 3D reconstructions) is essential to map patient-specific anatomy, guide precise screw placement, optimize craniocervical alignment, and reduce the risk of complications or revision surgery.

16. What surgical technique do you use for C1–C2 fusion: transarticular screws, Goel–Harms technique, etc.? Why it matters: Different techniques have different complication profiles and fusion success rates.

17. Will a bone graft be used? If so, what type (autograft, allograft, synthetic, or stem cell-enhanced)? Why it matters: Autografts (from your own bone) have higher fusion rates, but stem cell–enhanced options may improve outcomes with less morbidity.

18. What kind of imaging will be done post-op to monitor healing and hardware position? Why it matters: Follow-up imaging (e.g., CT, X-rays) is essential to track fusion progress and catch hardware issues early.

19. Will my case be handled by you or a resident/fellow during surgery? Why it matters: You have a right to know who is performing each part of your surgery, especially in teaching hospitals.

20. What is your plan if intraoperative complications occur (e.g., vertebral artery injury, dural tear, instability)? Why it matters: Complication readiness is a key marker of surgical quality and safety.

Referral Challenges and Self-Referral

Patients seeking care for CCI often face major challenges when trying to access the right specialists. Traditional referrals from a patient's primary care physician or specialist can be difficult, and many local neurosurgeons only accept life-threatening conditions and may also not have the advanced, specialized training required to accurately diagnose and treat CCI.

However, patients should try to get a referral to a local neurosurgeon anyway, in addition to a neurosurgeon specializing in CCI, whether it is remote or an in-person consultation. In other words, many patients self-refer to a neurosurgeon who specializes in CCI by searching and booking remote or in person consultations.

Self-referral can help accelerate the diagnostic process, but preparation is essential. Each neurosurgeon has specific requirements, such as MRI of the brain or spine, dynamic CT, or flexion-extension and rotational imaging. It's crucial to confirm what is needed before booking.

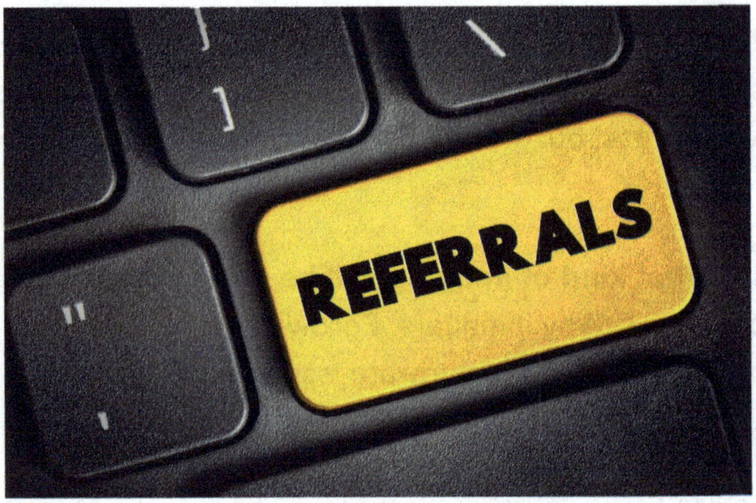

Having a trusted advocate, someone to help with administrative tasks involved in a self-referral like finding potential CCI neurosurgeons, asking patients and health provider for recommendations, filling out intake forms, submitting imaging and reports, arranging payments, and tracking communication, can make the process far less overwhelming.

Self-referral requires effort, but connecting with the right neurosurgeon who truly understands CCI can be life-changing.

How Many Neurosurgical Consultations Are Needed?

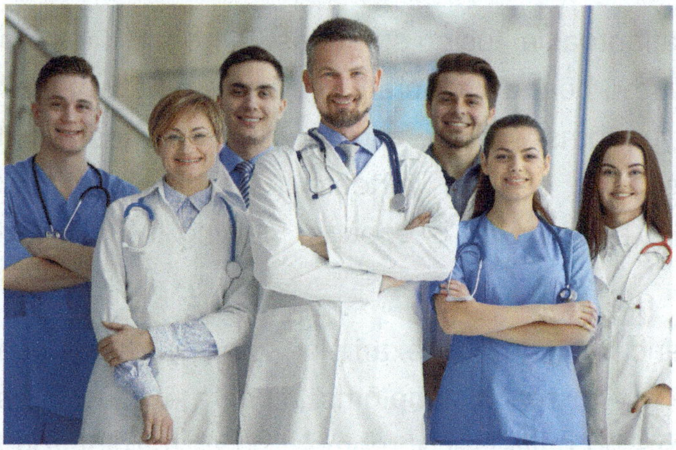

The number of neurosurgical consultations needed will vary depending on each patient's comfort level, personal situation, and financial resources.

Every neurosurgeon has their own approach, experience, and criteria for recommending surgery, so it's not uncommon for opinions to differ. One surgeon may suggest a more extensive procedure, such as an occiput-to-C2 fusion, while for the same patient, another surgeon may recommend a more limited C1–C2 fusion, stating the occiput to C1 instability is very minor and fusion of that area is not necessary. Some will only consider surgery when severe neurological symptoms, like gait issues or paralysis, are present, while others may recommend intervention when there is clear and severe instability causing significant symptoms and dysfunction.

Because not all neurosurgeons have the same level of training or experience in diagnosing and treating CCI, the type and quality of consultation matters. Remote consultations with CCI specialists can be an excellent way to access expert insights without the burden of travel. However, the level of detail provided can vary greatly. It can be helpful to speak with other patients who have consulted a particular surgeon, or request a nonspecific sample report from the surgeon's office to understand what kind of information is typically included in their remote consultation report.

Each consultation offers valuable information and perspective to help patients better understand their unique case. Some patients may feel confident after one opinion, while others find reassurance in seeking two, three or more. Remote reports from CCI specialists can also be presented to local neurosurgeons who perform AAF or CCF surgeries for an additional local opinion.

There is no set number of consultations that is "right" for everyone. The goal is for each patient to feel informed, confident, and supported in making the best possible decision for their care.

Controversies and Differences in Medical Opinions

Even with advances in craniocervical and atlantoaxial fusion surgeries, there's still a lot of disagreement among neurosurgeons about the best approach. For the same patient, one surgeon might recommend waiting until symptoms worsen, another might suggest a full fusion from the skull (occiput) to the second cervical vertebra (C2), while a third neurosurgeon may believe a more limited C1–C2 fusion is enough, viewing the occiput-to-C1 degree of instability as unnecessary.

There's also debate around certain tests and imaging. For example, some surgeons use invasive cervical traction (ICT) before surgery to see if symptoms improve, while others don't believe it's necessary. Similarly, there's no universal agreement on how to interpret borderline imaging results, like measurements of angles or misalignment between bones, and whether these should lead to surgery.

These differences come down to varying beliefs about when to be cautious and when to move forward with surgery. Some surgeons may overlook subtle signs of instability, while others may be quicker to recommend surgery. This is why it's common and often helpful for patients to seek more than one opinion. However, hearing very different recommendations can also be confusing and overwhelming.

Ultimately, the decision to have surgery should be based on a combination of clear severe symptoms, imaging findings, clinical judgment, and the patient's individual needs. A personalized plan from a surgeon with experience in CCI is key. There's no one-size-fits-all answer, just the approach that's right for each patient.

Deciding Whether to Have Surgery

Deciding to undergo surgery is a significant and deeply personal decision. It requires careful thought and a clear understanding of both the potential benefits and the possible risks. While the hope for improvement is natural, it must be weighed against the realities of what surgery might involve. If a patient still has a reasonable level of function in their daily life, surgery may not always be the best option.

There are usually three main reasons to seek a neurosurgical consultation:

1. To receive a clear and accurate diagnosis
2. To determine whether the surgeon believes surgery is a suitable option, and
3. Once all the information is available, to decide whether to continue with conservative treatment, or to proceed with surgery.

It's important to remember that most neurosurgical procedures are elective, meaning they are not emergency, or life-saving operations. The decision ultimately rests with the patient, based on their current condition, lifestyle, values, and the level of risk they are comfortable accepting.

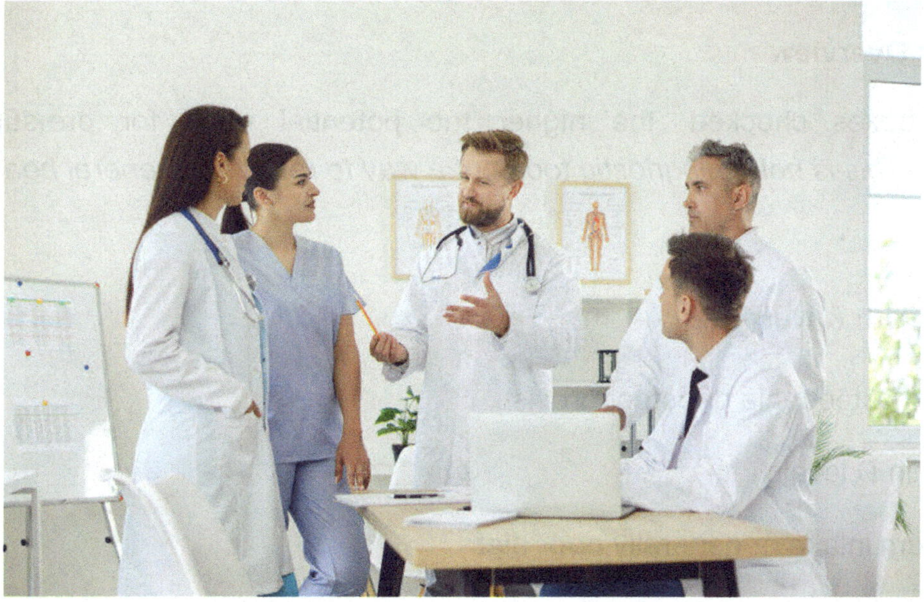

Once all the information is available, the patient can make an informed decision. For instance, if a person is currently functioning at 60%, is it worth undergoing a surgery that may only offer a 10% improvement in light of the chances of complications, such as a risk of fusion misalignment or even non-union (failure of the bones to heal properly)? The risks and benefits should be weighed by each patient, and each decision is very personal.

Each situation is unique, and every patient's tolerance for discomfort, risk, and uncertainty is different. What matters most is that the patient feels that they are fully supported, informed, have received all necessary investigations, examinations, and have a clear explanation of the surgeon's neurosurgical procedure (step by step) and have had the opportunity to carefully consider and weigh the potential benefits alongside the possible risks, in a way that aligns with their personal values, comfort level, and quality of life.

Personal Risk Factors Assessment for Craniocervical Fusion Surgery

This assessment outlines commonly recognized health factors that may increase the risk of complications or slower healing following craniocervical fusion surgery (including occipitocervical and atlantoaxial fusion). It is meant to help patients and care teams discuss how to reduce risk before surgery.

Risk Factor Overview

The more boxes checked, the higher the potential need for pre-surgical health optimization. *This is not a diagnostic tool, but a way to reflect on general health status.*

Bone Health & Nutrition

☐ Diagnosed osteopenia or osteoporosis

☐ Low vitamin D levels

☐ Low calcium intake or generally poor diet

☐ Weak bones on a bone density scan (DEXA)

💊 Medications & Substances

□ Regular use of NSAIDs (e.g., ibuprofen, naproxen)

□ Regular use of oral antihistamines (e.g., Benadryl, Claritin, Zyrtec)

□ Use of H2 blockers for heartburn (e.g., Pepcid, Zantac)

□ Use of steroids or corticosteroids (e.g., prednisone)

□ Regular use of alcohol

□ Regular use of THC (cannabis/marijuana)

🩺 Medical Conditions

□ Diagnosed connective tissue disorder (e.g., Ehlers-Danlos Syndrome)

□ Autoimmune disease (e.g., lupus, rheumatoid arthritis)

□ Diabetes (Type 1 or Type 2)

□ Chronic infections such as Hepatitis B, Hepatitis C, HIV, or Epstein-Barr virus (EBV)

□ History of Lyme disease or other tick-borne illness

□ Elevated inflammatory markers (e.g., CRP, ESR)

□ Abnormal blood work (e.g., RBC count, low hemoglobin, CBC abnormalities)

⚖️ Lifestyle & General Health

□ Smoking or nicotine use

□ Overweight or obese (high BMI)

□ Low physical activity, deconditioning, or mostly bedridden

□ Older age (especially over 65)

💬 How to Interpret This List

This list is a reflection tool. The more boxes checked, the more important it may be to work with healthcare providers to strengthen health before surgery. These factors do not mean surgery should be avoided, but may raise the risk of slower healing, reduced fusion, or complications.

✅ Ways to Potentially Lower Risk

- Improve diet, especially vitamin D, calcium, and protein
- Ask providers about tapering NSAIDs, steroids, or other high-risk medications
- Work on controlling blood sugar, autoimmune conditions, and inflammation
- Begin pre-surgery rehab or gentle movement, if approved by a doctor
- Screen and treat for bone health, infections or immune conditions if relevant

⚠️ Disclaimer

This guide is not a validated clinical scoring tool and has not been tested in formal research. It is provided for educational purposes only, to support conversations with healthcare providers. Future research may help confirm which personal risk factors most affect outcomes after craniocervical fusion surgery. Always consult a qualified medical professional before making decisions about treatment, medication, or surgery.

Chapter 2 Summary

This chapter empowers patients to take an active role in selecting a neurosurgeon and preparing for one of the most important medical decisions in their lives.

- Understanding the history and purpose of craniocervical fusion helps patients recognize why choosing the right surgeon is so critical.
- Caregiver support plays an essential role during consultations, in preparing for surgery, throughout the hospital stay, and during recovery.
- There are 10 key qualities to look for in a neurosurgeon, including experience, clear communication, thorough pre- and post-surgery assessment, structured aftercare, and referral to a CCF-expert physiotherapist.
- Referrals may not always be straightforward; in some cases, self-referral is necessary to reach the right specialist.
- It is common and often beneficial for patients to seek more than one consultation before making a surgical decision.
- Differences in medical opinions are expected; hearing multiple perspectives can help patients make a more balanced and confident choice.
- The decision to proceed with surgery requires weighing potential benefits against each patient's personal risk factors and readiness.

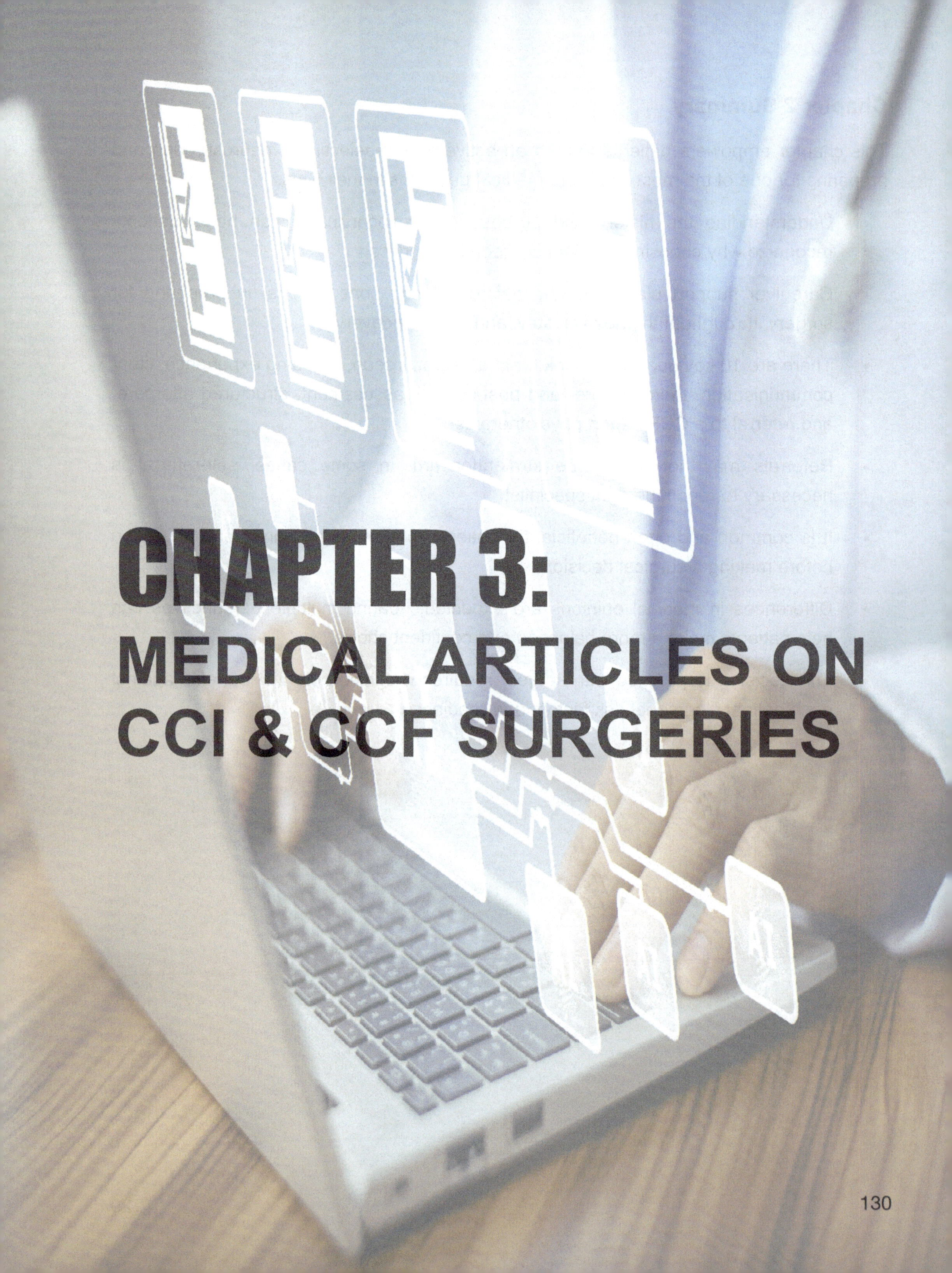

CHAPTER 3:
MEDICAL ARTICLES ON CCI & CCF SURGERIES

Introduction

This chapter includes short summaries of relevant case studies, systematic medical reviews, meta-analyses, and medical papers. In layman's terms, **systematic reviews** mean when medical researchers carefully look at all the good-quality studies that have been done on a certain treatment and combine the findings from all of them; meaning instead of just looking at one study, they look at *all of them* to get the full picture.

On the other hand, **meta-analysis**, which is the gold standard for evidence in evidence-based medicine, is when they take the numbers from those studies and combine them to see the overall results; kind of like averaging everything out, except these numbers help experts decide what works and what doesn't.

These studies provide an overview of congenital (from birth), traumatic (from injury), inflammatory (like arthritis), and infectious causes of CCI, specifically atlantoaxial (C1-C2) and atlanto-occipital (skull to C1) instability.

This chapter has been written to help patients better understand how different patients have experienced and managed these conditions, as well as recent advances and trends in the diagnosis and treatment of craniocervical junction disorders.

Reading these reviews may help patients make informed choices about when to see a neurosurgeon and what type of neurosurgeon experience is necessary, feel more confident and empowered in their healthcare, understand how symptoms and severity can vary from person to person, and be more prepared when speaking with doctors. However, not every case will match a patient's situation.

If reading these reviews feels overwhelming, causes unnecessary stress, or makes things more confusing, it's highly recommended to stop reading the reviews or skip this section entirely. These reviews are meant to support and not replace professional medical advice. If this chapter doesn't feel helpful, simply move on to the next.

Trigger Warning: Reading these medical reviews may cause patients unnecessary stress or make things more confusing. It's completely okay to skip this chapter.

The following summary of reviews will only cover some of the root causes of CCI in order for this chapter not to be too long. Medically reported root causes of CCI are included as follows:

1. Trauma-related (acquired instability) such as motor vehicle accidents, falls from height, sports injury or blunt force trauma such as assault.
2. Present at birth (congenital) such as Down syndrome, and more recently identified in the last couple of decades, Ehlers-Danlos Syndrome (EDS).
3. Chronic Inflammatory Diseases (acquired) such as rheumatoid arthritis or ankylosing spondylitis.
4. Infections (acquired) such as Grisel's Syndrome, Tuberculous Spondylitis (Pott's Disease) or Osteomyelitis.
5. Cancer (acquired).

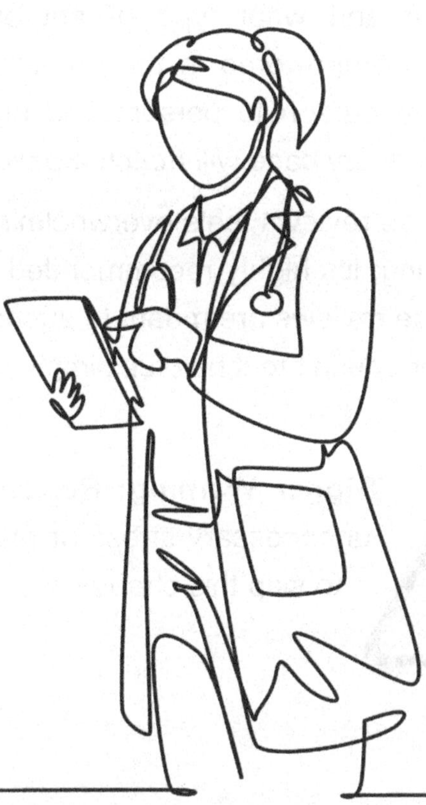

Medical Studies: Benefits and Risks of CCF Surgery

Occipitocervical Fusion (OCF) vs. Atlantoaxial Fusion (AAF)

A study in 2020 looked at **96 patients**, most of whom were older adults with an average age of 79, who had serious upper cervical spine injuries. These kinds of injuries are more common as people live longer and stay more active in their senior years.

Doctors used two main types of surgery to stabilize the neck: atlantoaxial fusion (AAF), and occipitocervical fusion (OCF). Both surgeries provide more stability to the upper cervical spine, but OCF limits neck movement much more than AAF.

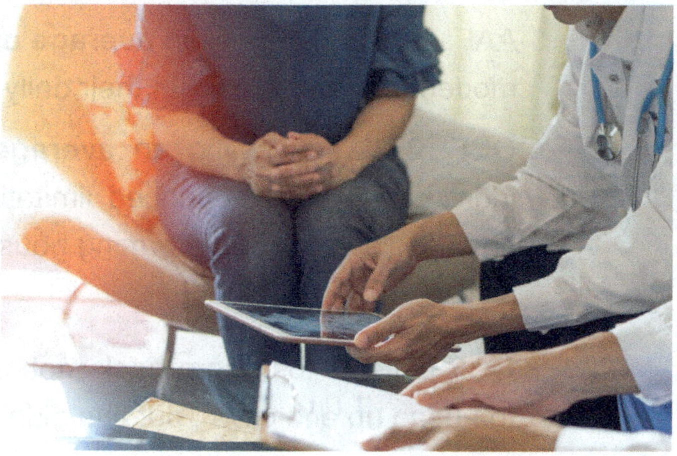

Patients who had OCF tended to have more health problems (i.e. comorbidities) than those who had AAF. Common health problems in these patients included osteoporosis or osteopenia (i.e. weaker bones that may not hold screws or plates well), heart disease or high blood pressure (which can raise the risk of surgery), diabetes (which slows wound healing and increases infection risk), lung diseases like COPD (which can make recovery and anesthesia harder), memory problems like dementia (which can make rehab and follow-up care harder), degenerative spine disease (where other parts of the spine are already stiff or weak).

These conditions can affect healing, and increase the risk of complications. OCF is often preferred for patients with more severe injuries, poor bone quality, or multiple health issues, because it provides more immediate stability.

Of the 96 patients with an average of 79 years of age, 52 had AAF and 44 had OCF surgery. All were followed at least 6 months after surgery. The surgery outcomes reported by the patients were as follows:

- **Both groups reported mild pain after surgery (scale 0 = no pain to 10 = worst pain).**
    - AAF: average pain score of 2.0 reflecting mild pain
    - OCF: average pain score of 2.9 reflecting mild pain
- **Neck Disability Index Score (NDI)**

  NDI is a standardized questionnaire to measure how much a person's neck pain is affecting their daily activities and overall quality of life. It includes 10 sections, each addressing a specific function such as pain intensity, personal care, lifting, reading, headaches, concentration, work, driving, sleeping, and recreation.

    - AAF: 21% suggesting an **average of mild disability**, meaning that neck pain moderately interferes with their daily activities like reading, driving, or lifting.
    - OCF: 37% suggesting an **average of moderate disability**, meaning the individual likely experienced limitations in daily activities, such as working, driving, sleeping, or performing household tasks, due to neck pain.
- **Loss of Neck Movement**
    - OCF patients lost more neck motion (up to 25 degrees), especially bending the head up and down, but this didn't make daily life harder for most.
- **Complications After Surgery**
    - Infection:
        - AAF = 7.7% of patients
        - OCF = 4.5% of patients
    - Revision surgery:
        - AAF = 17.3% of patients
        - OCF = 13.6% of patients
- **No fatal outcomes were reported.**
- **Recovery Over Time**
    - Patients who were followed for a longer time tended to feel better and had improved disability scores, meaning that people often adjust and heal well over time, even if recovery starts off slowly.

Fusion Complications

A study from 2010 aimed to look at the rates of complications that happened during craniocervical fusions and to explore strategies that can help reduce these risks before and during surgery. The study analyzed **2,274 procedures** for complications. The most common issues during the surgery were related to problems with the following:

- **Surgical hardware (I.e. screw) failure, especially due to nonunion** (i.e. when the bone graft does not grow and heal properly). These problems occurred in:
    - 7% of occipitocervical fusion surgeries
    - 6.7% of atlantoaxial fusion surgeries
- **Damage to the vertebral artery** 1.3% to 4.1% of surgeries involving C1-C2 screws, especially when the artery was higher than normal
- **Tears in the protective covering around the spinal cord** (dural tears)
- **Infections at the wound site**

Despite these risks, occipitocervical and atlantoaxial fusion surgeries can be done safely with low chances of serious complications if there is careful surgical planning.

Safety is improved when doctors properly assess each patient's anatomy before surgery and are well-prepared to handle all potential problems during the procedure.

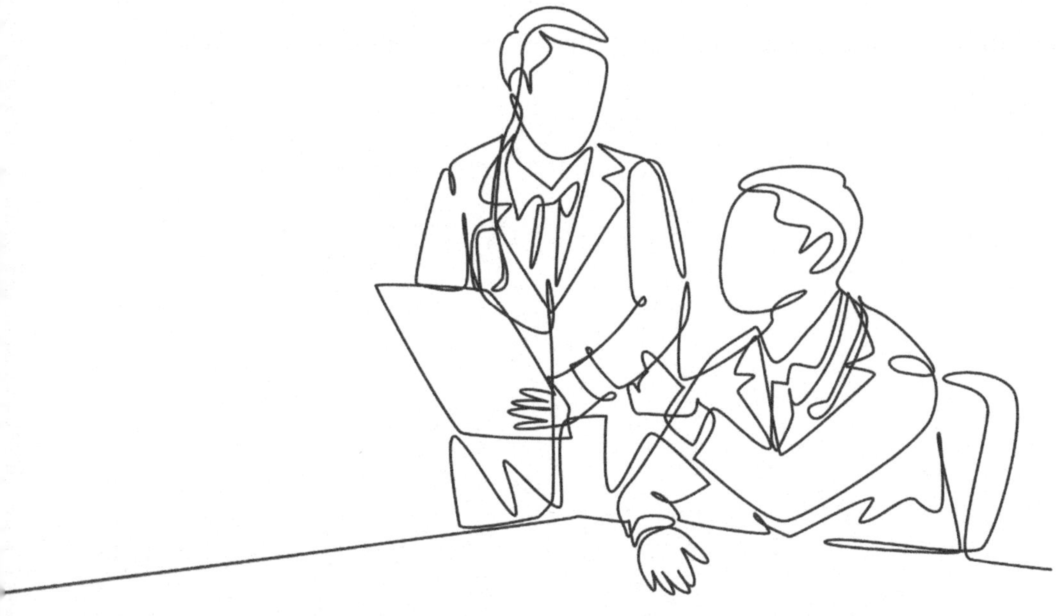

C1-C2 Fusion Surgery Complications

In a very small study of 20 patients who had undergone atlantoaxial (C1-C2) fusion surgery, there were no apparent complications during the surgery itself.

Revision Surgery:

Two out of twenty patients (i.e. 10%) needed revision surgery to redo their fusions within 12 months after the operation.

Trip and Fall:

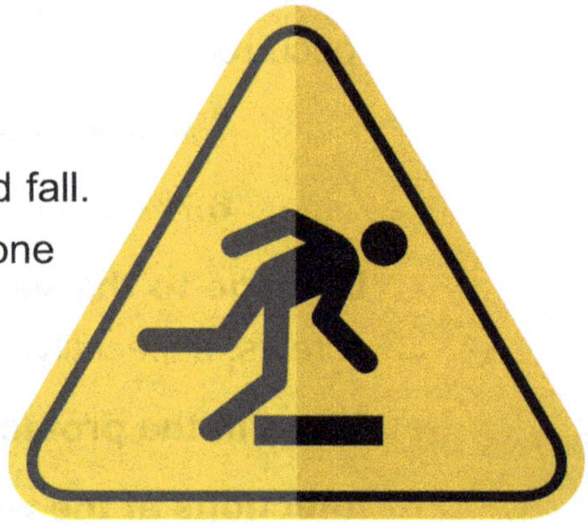

One patient required revision after experiencing a trip and fall. Before the fall, a CT scan showed early signs of bone growth but this growth was lost after the fall.

This highlights that the fusion process is slow and can take at least 12 months or more to fully stabilize in these patients.

Hardware Failure:

The other patient showed successful bone fusion between the C1 and C2 vertebrae on a CT scan six months post-surgery. However, a broken screw at the C1 level was detected on a follow-up scan at 12 months.

This indicates that even when the bone fusion is successful, the mechanical stresses applied to the C1 area can be significant enough to cause metal hardware breakage. This risk is heightened when factors like osteopenia (weaker bones) and smaller bone size can lead to a higher chance of fusion failure, especially in patients with rotational instability.

Sample of CCF Complications Rates

- Suboccipital numbness (i.e. back of head) in 16.8% to 50% of patients, which typically goes away over time.
- Screw misplacement (24.5%) (i.e. meaning screws are incorrectly positioned during surgery and can cause nerve damage, misalignment, and hardware failure.)
- Injury to the vertebral artery (1.2% to 8.2%)
- Neurological problems (0.2% to 3.7%) e.g. pain, weakness, dizziness, numbness, swallowing difficulty, and balance problems.
- Failed fusion (0.2%)
- Tears in the dural covering of the spinal cord (0.3%)
- Screws breaking out at the atlanto-axial joint (0.4%) (i.e. meaning the screws came loose or pulled out from the bone where they were placed.)
  - Note: Screws can come loose or break out at the C1-C2 joint because of
    - weak bone quality
    - incorrect screw placement
    - too much movement before healing
    - repeated stress on the screws, or
    - if the bones don't fuse properly after surgery.
- Screw fractures (0.8%) (i.e. "hardware failure" meaning the screws themselves actually broke or snapped while still inside the bone.)
- Infections (0.5%) (i.e. infections can cause the need for surgery (to take out the infection), weaken bone, loosen screws, and delay healing after surgery.)
- Suboccipital neuralgia (0.1%)
- Death (0.1%)

Based on the CCF Complications Reported, to provide a rough estimate of complication rates per 1,000 patients may be projected at:

- Suboccipital numbness (which typically goes away over time): 168 to 500 patients
- Screw misplacement (i.e. screws incorrectly positioned): 245 patients
- Vertebral artery injury: 12 to 82 patients
- Neurological problems: 2 to 37 patients
- Failed fusion: 2 patients
- Dural tears: 3 patients
- Screws breaking out at atlanto-axial joint: 4 patients
- Screw fractures: 8 patients
- Infections: 5 patients
- Suboccipital neuralgia: 1 patient
- Death: 1 patient

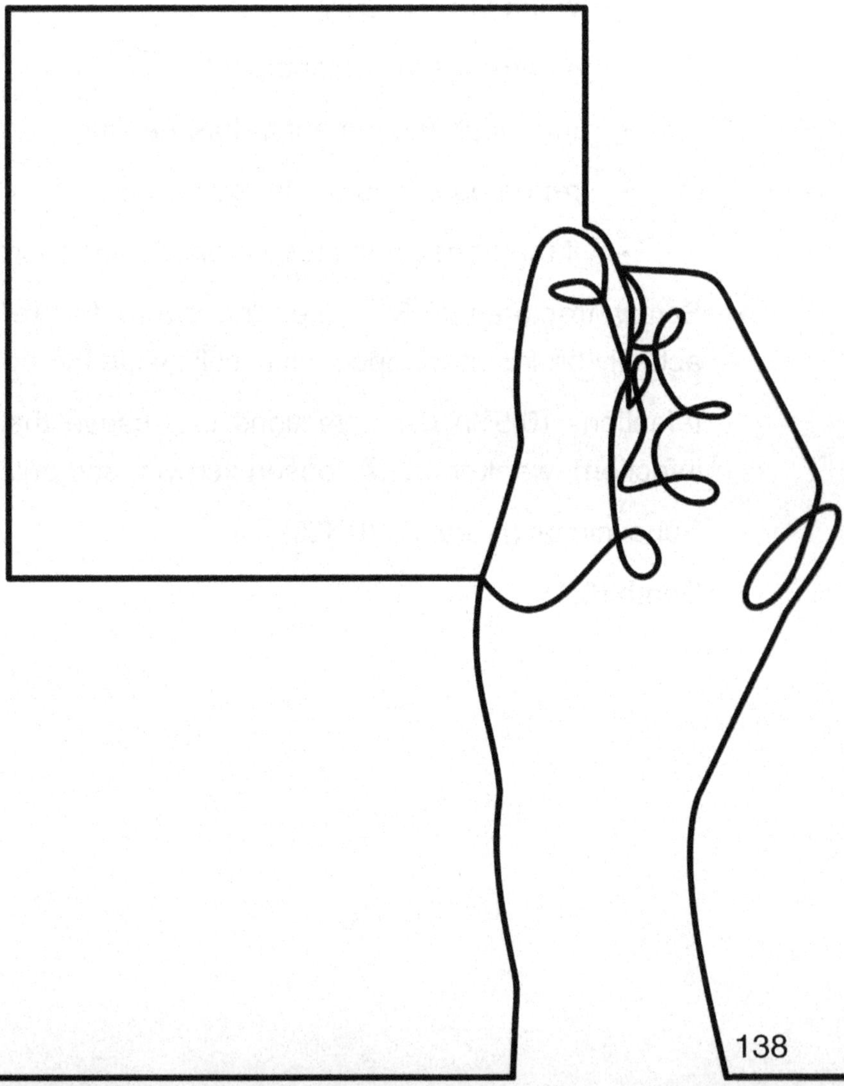

Traumatic Atlanto-Occipital Dislocations

Understanding Traumatic Atlanto-Occipital Dislocation
— *A rare but life-threatening neck injury*

Traumatic Atlanto-Occipital Dislocation (TAOD) is a rare and serious condition where the skull becomes dislocated from the top of the spine, usually after major high-velocity trauma such as car accidents, falls, or sports injuries. It can cause severe neurological damage or death if not treated quickly.

A review of 17 studies, covering **341 patients** from the early 1990s to 2020, found that 119 patients (35%) died due to the severity of the injury.

A key issue highlighted was delayed diagnosis in 22 cases (6.5%). TAOD wasn't recognized early, often because initial CT scans or X-rays didn't reveal the injury. This delay worsened the condition and postponed critical treatment.

Later use of MRI scans proved much more effective, clearly showing ligament damage and the extent of dislocation.

6.5% Delayed AOD diagnosis because

CT Scans or X-rays images failed to

reveal any signs of damage or problems.

Medical Imaging

Imaging is essential for identifying TAOD and guiding treatment.

CT scans help assess skull-to-spine alignment using specific measures like the Basion-Dens Interval (BDI), Basion-Axial Interval (BAI), Power Ratio, and Condyle-C1 Interval (CCI).

MRI is especially valuable for detecting soft tissue and ligament injuries that might be missed on other scans.

Early and accurate diagnosis, especially with CT scans and MRI can make a life-saving difference in managing this rare but dangerous injury.

Below is a detailed summary of the radiological findings, organized by the key measurements:

- **Basion-Dens Interval (BDI):** An abnormal BDI, typically greater than 1.4 cm, was found in over 80% of patients with TAOD. A BDI of 16 mm or more was associated with worse outcomes, including fatalities, highlighting its value in identifying severe dislocations.
- **Basion-Axial Interval (BAI):** Used alongside the BDI, an abnormal BAI often pointed to severe instability. In most cases, at least one of these two measurements was abnormal, reinforcing the importance of using them together in evaluation.
- **Power Ratio:** This measurement assesses alignment between the skull and spine. Over 50% of patients with TAOD had a Power ratio greater than 1, which generally indicated significant displacement. It was particularly helpful when other markers were borderline or unclear.
- **Prevertebral Hematoma** (when blood collects in the space just in front of the spine) **& Retropharyngeal Swelling** (behind the throat)**:** These soft tissue signs were commonly observed in imaging and helped flag potential TAOD. Prevertebral hematomas were especially frequent and strongly suggested upper cervical injury, although retropharyngeal swelling showed more variability.
- **Other Findings:** Base of skull (occipital condyle fractures) occurred in about 50% of the cases. C1-C2 subluxations (misalignments), ligament injuries, and fractures were also frequently associated. MRI was essential in detecting ligamentous injuries missed by CT scans or X-rays, especially in patients with ongoing symptoms despite normal early scans.

The review concluded that while X-rays and CT scans were commonly used, they sometimes failed to diagnose TAOD, with MRI has become essential for accurate diagnosis in certain cases. The variability in diagnostic criteria across studies reflects the complexity of diagnosing TAOD and the need for standardized methods to improve patient outcomes.

Patient Symptoms

Some patients initially *showed no symptoms*, making it difficult for doctors to diagnose TAOD early on. Symptoms might have appeared later, but the exact timing isn't clear.

Treatment

When it came to treatment, surgery was the most common approach. About 57% of patients underwent surgery, which usually involved occipito-cervical fusion. For patients whose condition wasn't as severe, non-surgical treatments were considered. Around 11% of patients were treated non-surgically. These patients often used a neck collar, a halo vest, or Crutchfield tongs to stabilize the neck. These devices are designed to keep the neck in a fixed position, allowing the dislocation to heal while preventing further damage to the spine.

The decision to perform surgery typically depended on the severity of the injury and the symptoms the patient experienced. Patients with significant neck pain, weakness, or neurological issues were more likely to need surgery. In some cases, patients without symptoms may still require surgery if their scans show a serious dislocation of the skull or instability in the spine.

Conclusion

This review highlights the importance of early diagnosis and treatment in patients with TAOD. This condition can be fatal if not diagnosed and treated quickly. Imaging tests, such as CT and MRI scans, are essential tools for detecting this injury early. While children are especially vulnerable, most patients require surgery to stabilize the neck, though some less severe cases can be managed with non-surgical treatments like halo vests or neck collars. Early and appropriate treatment can make a significant difference in recovery and reduce the risk of long-term disability.

Atlanto-Axial Dislocations

This summary highlights a 2014 review of the diagnosis and treatment of atlantoaxial dislocations, which examined 112 articles **over almost 50 years**, that were published between 1966 and 2014.

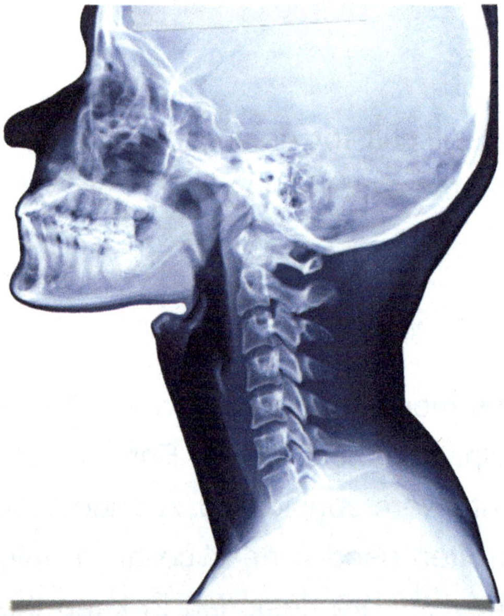

Atlantoaxial dislocation (AAD) is a condition where there is instability or misalignment between the first two vertebrae in the neck (C1 (atlas) and C2 (axis)). This joint is crucial for head rotation and overall neck mobility. When the ligaments supporting this joint are damaged or weakened, the bones can shift, potentially leading to neurological complications.

AAD can be caused by trauma, congenital, or inflammatory diseases. Symptoms range from mild neck pain to severe neurological issues such as weakness, numbness, difficulty breathing, or paralysis. AAD requires close monitoring.

To diagnose AAD, imaging plays a central role. A key diagnostic tool is the Atlantodental Interval (ADI), which measures the space between the dens (part of C2) and the ring of C1. An increased ADI indicates instability. For adults, an ADI greater than 3 mm and for children, greater than 5 mm suggests a dislocation. Additional surgical diagnostic criteria include:

- ADI exceeding normal limits (greater than 3 mm for adults, 5 mm for children)
- Disruption of the transverse or alar ligaments, visible on MRI
- Forward translation of C1 on C2
- Instability or abnormal movement identified through dynamic imaging (flexion and extension X-rays)
- Neurological symptoms caused by spinal cord compression
- Congenital conditions such as os odontoideum or dens hypoplasia

Surgical intervention is often recommended for AAD to prevent serious complications, including respiratory failure and irreversible neurological damage. Surgery is typically advised when instability is confirmed and symptoms are present, such as:

- Symptomatic dislocation with signs of spinal cord compression
- Asymptomatic cases with severe instability or an ADI greater than 5 mm in adults or 4 mm in children, especially when imaging shows progressive instability or signs of neurological decline
- Congenital or rheumatologic conditions such as Down syndrome or rheumatoid arthritis, which increase the risk of sudden deterioration

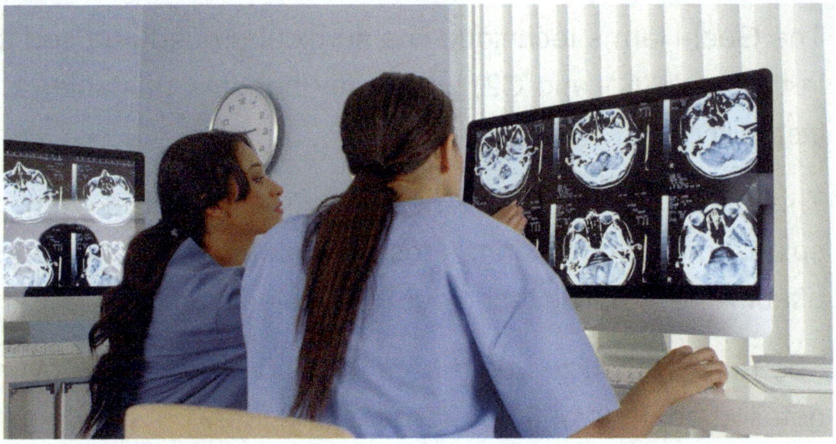

In some mild cases, a neck brace may be used instead of surgery, particularly if the dislocation is recent or not causing significant instability.

Surgical options primarily aim to stabilize the C1-C2 joint through fusion techniques. These surgeries are generally performed when the instability poses a risk of further neurological injury or if conservative treatments like bracing are ineffective.

Before surgical fixation, traction may be applied to reduce the dislocation. This process involves gradually applying weight to stretch the surrounding tissues and align the C1 and C2 vertebrae. Successful reduction is indicated when the ADI decreases to normal levels (<3 mm in adults, <5 mm in children). If reduction is not successful, surgical techniques like anterior decompression may be needed in addition to posterior fusion to fully decompress the spinal cord and restore alignment.

Atlantoaxial dislocation is a rare but serious condition that can lead to severe complications if untreated. Early diagnosis through imaging, particularly measuring the ADI and assessing ligament integrity is crucial. Surgical intervention is often necessary when instability is present and symptoms are significant, aiming to prevent further neurological damage and ensure spinal stability.

The choice of surgical technique varies based on the severity of the dislocation, the patient's anatomy, and the presence of any congenital or inflammatory conditions. With appropriate treatment, the risk of long-term disability or death can be minimized, allowing for improved outcomes for affected patients.

Atlantoaxial Fusion Surgery

A Comprehensive Review of the Safety and Effectiveness of the Goel-Harms Technique

The following is a summary of the systematic review and meta-analysis titled Efficacy and Safety of Goel-Harms Technique in Upper Cervical Spine Surgery that was published in World Neurosurgery in 2022.

The Goel-Harms technique is a surgical procedure used to stabilize the top two vertebrae in the neck (C1 and C2) when they become unstable, a condition known as atlantoaxial instability.

This instability can cause neck pain, restricted movement, and, in more serious cases, spinal cord compression. A recent systematic review and study focused on the safety and effectiveness of this technique, particularly in patients from the Asian population.

The review analyzed data from 86 studies, covering over 4,200 patients, and included a detailed analysis of **53 patients** who underwent the surgery between 2010 and 2018. The results showed that the Goel-Harms technique had a very high success rate, with 98.13% of patients achieving successful fusion, meaning their C1 and C2 vertebrae healed together properly. Patients also reported significant improvements in neck function, pain levels, and overall quality of life.

98.13% of patients achieved successful fusion

Neck Disability Index

The Neck Disability Index (NDI), which assesses *how neck pain interferes with daily life*, showed a large decrease in disability, with most patients improving significantly. NDI dropped from:

- an average of 31.62 (+/- 11.05) before surgery (moderate to severe disability from neck pain)
- an average 8.68 (+/- 3.76) after surgery (much less pain and could do more in daily life). This shows that surgery helped most patients feel significantly better and improved their ability to function.

Pain Levels

Most patients reported major pain relief. Pain levels measured by the Visual Analog Scale (VAS), went from:

- 4.85 (+/- 1.03) before surgery
- 1.02 (+/- 0.87) after surgery

This means that before surgery, patients rated their pain as moderate (about 5 out of 10 on the pain scale). After surgery, their pain dropped to about 1 out of 10, meaning most patients had very little pain afterward. This shows that the surgery provided major pain relief for most people.

Nerve and Spinal Cord Function

Patients regained better nerve function and comfort after surgery. Nerve and spinal cord function were evaluated using the Japanese Orthopaedic Association (JOA) score, which improved from:

- 13.20 (+/-3.96) to 15.2 (+/- 2.17) in patients who had spinal cord issues.

This means, for patients who had problems with their spinal cord or nerves, the surgery helped improve how well their nerves were working. Their JOA score, which measures nerve and spinal cord function, went up after surgery — from about 13 to 15 out of 17, showing better movement, feeling, and comfort. This means the surgery helped many patients regain some nerve function and reduce symptoms like numbness, weakness, or coordination problems.

Procedure Safety

The procedure was also relatively safe. Complications included:

- vertebral artery injury occurred in just 2.8% of cases
- issues with screw placement 5.8% of cases or nerve irritation in 6.1% of cases

The safest outcomes came from placing **transpedicular screws** through the more stable parts of the C1 and C2 bones, which also reduced blood loss. Importantly, the surgery could be performed using traditional methods, without advanced imaging tools, and still maintain a strong safety profile.

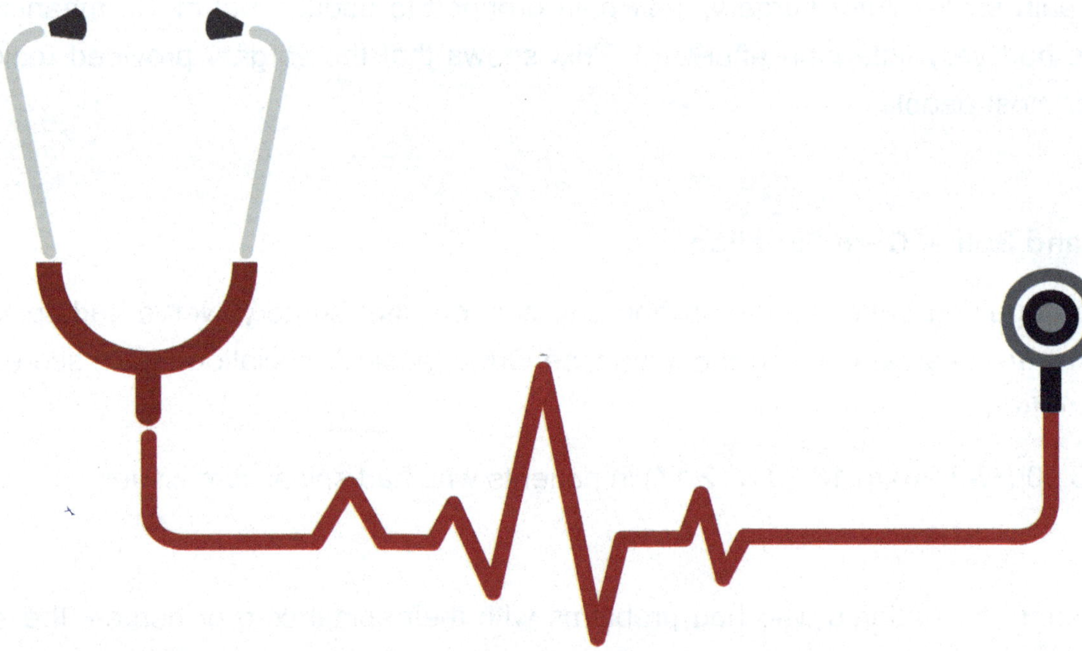

Down Syndrome and CCI

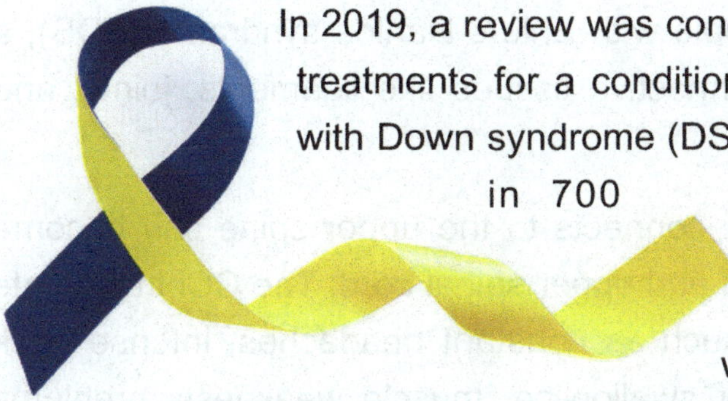

In 2019, a review was conducted by medical experts to evaluate surgical treatments for a condition called atlantoaxial instability (AAI) in people with Down syndrome (DS). DS is a genetic disorder that affects about 1 in 700 babies, causing developmental delays, physical differences, and other health issues. One common problem for people with DS is AAI, which is when the top two neck bones become unstable, potentially causing pain, stiffness, and nerve issues.

AAI affects roughly 12% to 20% of people with DS. When this happens, surgery is often recommended to stabilize the neck and protect the spinal cord. The surgery typically involves decompressing the spinal cord and using rods, screws, or wires to keep the bones in place. Sometimes, a fusion is done to help the bones heal together. However, surgery can be risky, and complications like infections, nerve damage, or the need for additional surgeries can occur.

The review analyzed existing studies to determine which surgical methods worked best for people with DS. It found that a combination of screws and rods had the highest success rates, leading to better healing of the bones and fewer complications compared to just using wires alone. However, it's important to note that treating AAI in people with DS is still controversial, as each person's anatomy is unique and delicate, which can make surgery more challenging.

The review also highlighted that more research is needed to improve surgical techniques and patient outcomes. While screws and rods appear to offer the best results, there's no one-size-fits-all solution, and the best treatment approach is still being debated.

While surgery can help improve stability and prevent further issues, there are risks involved. For the Down syndrome patient population with atlantoaxial instability, the use of screws and rods seems to provide the best outcomes so far, but ongoing research will help refine these methods and improve long-term results.

Outcomes of Occipito-Cervical Fusion in EDS Patients

CCI is a serious condition that can affect people with Ehlers-Danlos syndrome (EDS), a genetic disorder that weakens the body's connective tissues like ligaments, joints, and skin.

In people with EDS, the area where the skull connects to the upper spine can become unstable, leading to pressure on the brainstem and upper spinal cord. The CCI in patients can cause severe and disabling symptoms such as constant headaches, intense neck pain, dizziness, fainting, difficulty speaking or swallowing, muscle weakness, problems with balance, and even issues with memory and thinking clearly.

Some patients also have a condition called Chiari malformation or low-lying cerebellar tonsils (part of the brain), which can block the flow of cerebrospinal fluid (CSF) and make symptoms worse.

In this study, doctors wanted to see if a surgery called occipito-cervical fusion (OCF) could help patients with EDS who had severe symptoms of CCI and had not improved with non-surgical treatments like pain medication, neck braces, or physical therapy. The study included **53 adults with EDS** who had been living with these symptoms, on average, for about 12 years before being referred for surgery. Many of them had sudden onset of symptoms following events such as car accidents, childbirth, sports injuries, surgeries, or infections.

All 53 patients underwent OCF, which is a surgery that realigns the bones at the base of the skull and the top of the spine and fuses them together using special hardware and bone grafts to stabilize the area.

In 32 of these patients, the surgeons also performed decompression surgery to improve CSF flow because these individuals had Chiari malformation, low-lying tonsils, or narrowing in the skull opening (foramen magnum). Imaging studies, including MRI and CT scans, were used before surgery to confirm the diagnosis and determine who would benefit from the operation.

The results of the surgery were encouraging. Results were as follows:

Pain: Patients showed significant improvement in pain and neurological symptoms.

- Patients rated their headache and neck pain at an average of 4.3 out of 5 before surgery
- After surgery, patients rated their headache and neck pain dropped to an average of 3.3 out of 5.
- There was no meaningful difference in pain improvement between patients with Chiari or low-lying tonsils and those without these conditions.
- More than half of the patients, (52%) also reported that they were able to reduce their use of pain medication.

Daily Functioning: Functionally, patients experienced improvements in their ability to manage everyday activities. Patient's median Karnofsky Performance Scores, which measures how well someone can carry out daily tasks,

- 50 before surgery to 60 after surgery

Neurological Symptoms: Neurological symptoms also improved across the board. Many patients reported fewer issues with dizziness, nausea, fainting, speech problems, difficulty concentrating, and vertigo. There were also reductions in symptoms like numbness, arm weakness, and poor coordination.

Mental Fatigue: A test measuring mental fatigue, called the Wood Mental Fatigue Inventory, showed that patients' average score improved from 23 to 18 after surgery.

Opinion on the Surgery: 94% of the patients said they would choose to undergo the surgery again if faced with the same situation. Overall, 75% of patients reported general improvement in their condition after surgery. Only 17% reported that their overall condition had worsened, mainly due to other health problems common in people with EDS, such as fatigue, mast cell activation syndrome, TMJ dysfunction, and dysautonomia (problems with automatic body functions like heart rate and blood pressure).

Procedure Safety: While the surgery was generally safe, a small number of patients experienced complications. Four patients needed follow-up surgery for wound healing problems, and 12 underwent other unrelated surgeries during the study period, such as treatment for tethered spinal cord or fluid pressure issues in the brain.

How hEDS Patients Often Face a Chain of Serious Conditions

Connective tissue disorders (CTDs) are a group of conditions that affect the body's connective tissues, the parts that hold everything together, like joints, skin, and organs. These disorders can lead to a wide range of problems, especially with movement, the immune system, and the nervous system. One of the most common CTDs is called hypermobile Ehlers-Danlos Syndrome (hEDS). People with hEDS often have very flexible joints, chronic pain, and may also suffer from conditions that affect how their body moves, digests food, and responds to infections or injuries.

The study reviewed **717 patients** referred to a neurosurgical center between 2014 and 2023. Patients had either a confirmed or suspected connective tissue disorder (CTD) or related symptoms. About 64% were diagnosed with hypermobile Ehlers-Danlos syndrome (hEDS). Most patients were women, with an average age of 37.

The study found that patients with hEDS were much more likely than others to have certain additional conditions, including:

- Dysautonomia (when the nervous system doesn't regulate body functions properly, like heart rate or blood pressure)
- POTS (Postural Orthostatic Tachycardia Syndrome) (a condition causing rapid heartbeat when standing)
- MCAD (Mast Cell Activation Disorder) (causes allergic-type reactions)
- Gastroparesis (delayed emptying of the stomach)
- Tethered Cord Syndrome (TCS) (spinal cord is abnormally attached inside the spine)
- GERD (acid reflux)
- Hypothyroidism, small fiber neuropathy, and chronic fatigue

About 85% of patients in the study ended up having some type of surgery. For many, the reason was due to craniocervical instability which may be especially serious because it may press on the brainstem or spinal cord.

The most common surgeries included:

- Craniocervical Fusion (CCF) – to stabilize the neck and skull
- Posterior Fossa Decompression (PFD) – to relieve pressure on the brain for patients with Chiari Malformation Type I (CMI)
- Tethered Cord Release (TCR) – to fix Tethered Cord Syndrome
- Other surgeries like cerebrospinal fluid (CSF) leak repairs, shunts, and removal of bone growths were also done.

Among the people with hEDS, 73% needed CCF surgery. This shows that craniocervical instability is a serious issue in this group.

One interesting finding was that many people with hEDS also had POTS and MCAD: an **"hEDS Trio"**. In fact, about one-third of hEDS patients had all three conditions at once. These three often come together and may be connected in how they affect the body's systems. The study found that people with these conditions were more likely to need surgeries like CCF and TCR, showing how serious the symptoms can be when these conditions overlap.

The study compared people with hEDS to those without connective tissue disorders and found important differences:

- People with hEDS were more likely to have multiple health issues at once.
- They were also more likely to need complex surgeries and not just one, but often combinations of two or three.
- Those without hEDS had fewer immune or nervous system issues but still needed surgery for structural brain or spine problems, like CMI.

This study helps highlight a few important things:

1. People with hEDS often have more than just joint problems. They can also suffer from serious neurological, digestive, and immune system conditions.
2. Many of these health problems can overlap, which makes diagnosis and treatment more complicated.
3. Surgery is often needed, especially when the bones in the neck or skull are unstable or when the spinal cord is under pressure.
4. More research is needed to understand why these conditions happen together and how to treat them better.

This was the first study of its kind to closely examine how people with connective tissue disorders, especially hEDS, often face multiple, overlapping health challenges that can affect daily life.

The study found that hEDS often comes with other health problems involving the nerves, muscles, immune system, and blood pressure. Many of these issues may require surgery. Understanding these connections can lead to earlier diagnosis and better care. For doctors, it highlights the need to look at the whole patient, not just one problem at a time.

It is important to note that the study focused on severe cases at a surgical center, and it may not reflect every hEDS patient. Ongoing research may help improve how physicians recognize and treat these complex conditions.

Dysautonomia Symptoms: Does Craniocervical Fusion Help?

Dysautonomia Outcomes After Craniocervical Fusion in Non-EDS Patients with CCI

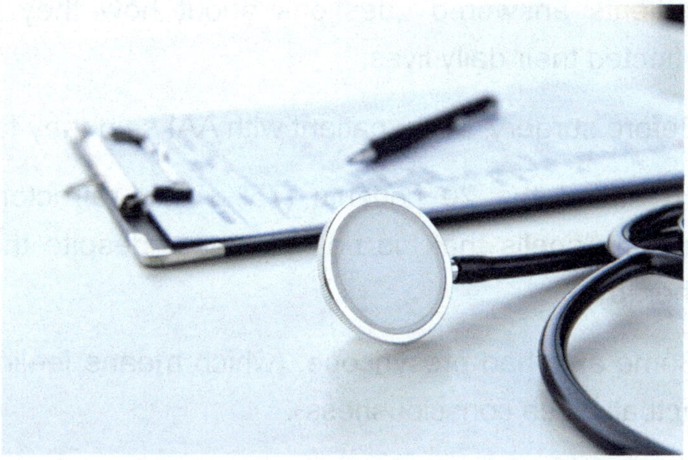

A small study from 2021 looked at 33 adults who had a condition called Chiari malformation and abnormalities in the craniocervical junction. These patients had craniocervical fusion (CCF), and some also had extra work done to relieve pressure on the brainstem.

The researchers checked for symptoms like headaches, neck and shoulder pain, dizziness or feeling like the room is spinning, trouble thinking clearly and problems with automatic body functions (called dysautonomia).

Before surgery, over half of the patients had dysautonomia symptoms. After surgery, many patients reported that their dysautonomia symptoms improved; however, the improvement wasn't strong enough to prove for certain that the surgery caused the change. The study had concluded that surgery might help with dysautonomia, but we need more research to know for sure.

Before CCF surgery, 18 patients with dysautonomia reported the following outcomes after CCF surgery:

- 6 patients reported complete improvement (~ 33% of the patients)
- 8 patients reported partial improvement (~ 44.4%)
- 3 patients reported unchanged dysautonomia symptoms (~ 17%)
- 0 patients reported new or worse dysautonomia symptoms

Dysautonomia Outcomes After Atlantoaxial Fusion in Patients with Connective Tissue Disorders

In 2021, a small study looked at **20 patients** who had connective tissue disorders and a problem called atlantoaxial instability (AAI). All of these patients had surgery to fix and stabilize the top two bones in their neck (called C1 and C2). Before and after surgery, the patients answered questions about how they were feeling and how their symptoms affected their daily lives.

Before surgery, every patient with AAI said they felt lightheaded.

15 out of the 20 patients (75%) had refractory syncope (meaning they experienced fainting spells that did not get better despite the best medical treatments and physical therapy).

Some also had presyncope, (which means feeling like they were about to faint but didn't actually lose consciousness).

Postoperatively, subjects reported an improvement in lightheadedness, presyncope, and syncope, and a *significant* improvement in the frequency of other symptoms related to autonomic function, such as nausea, exercise intolerance, palpitations, tremors, heat intolerance, gastroesophageal reflux, and sleep apnea.

While the results in this study show some promise, more research is needed to confirm how well this surgery helps patients with these conditions.

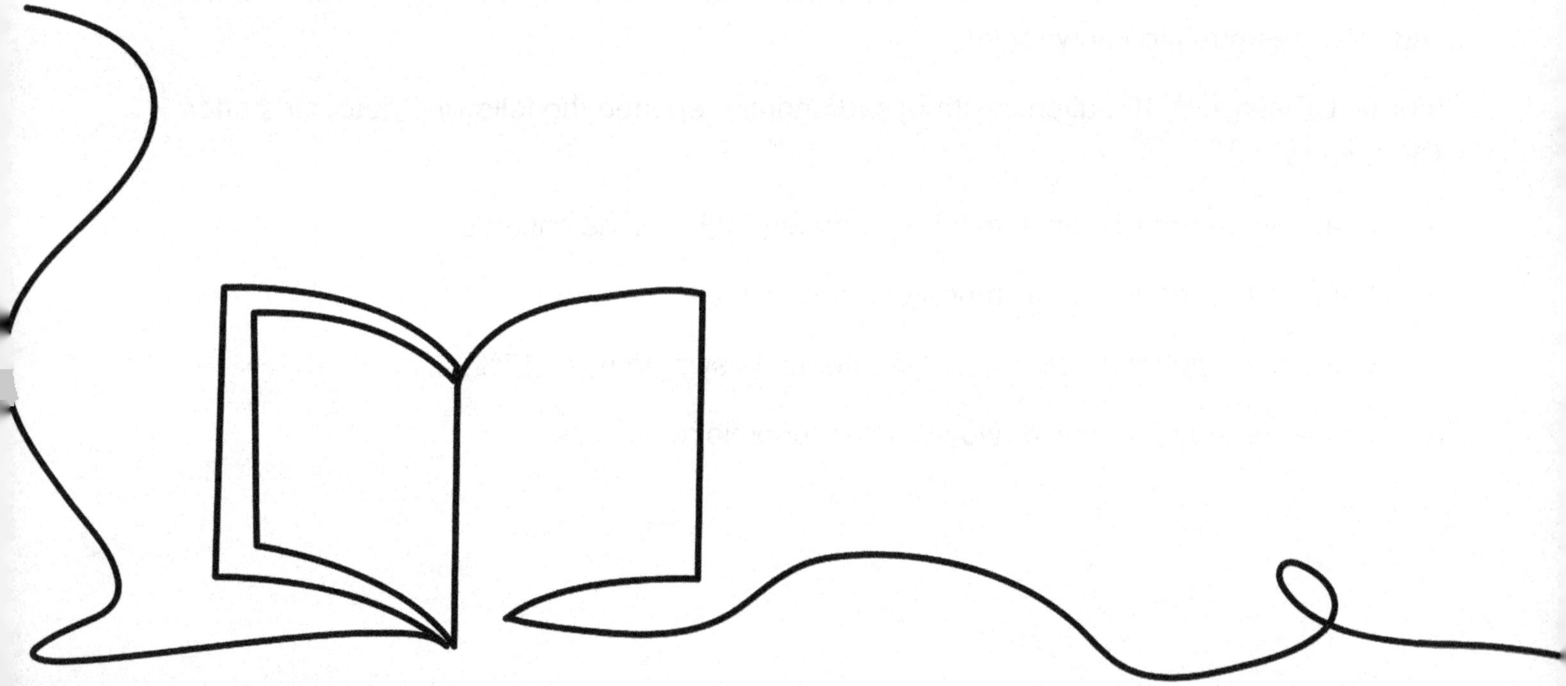

Rheumatoid Arthritis and CCI

Rheumatoid arthritis (RA) is a chronic autoimmune disease where the immune system mistakenly attacks the joints, causing chronic inflammation, pain, and potential joint damage.

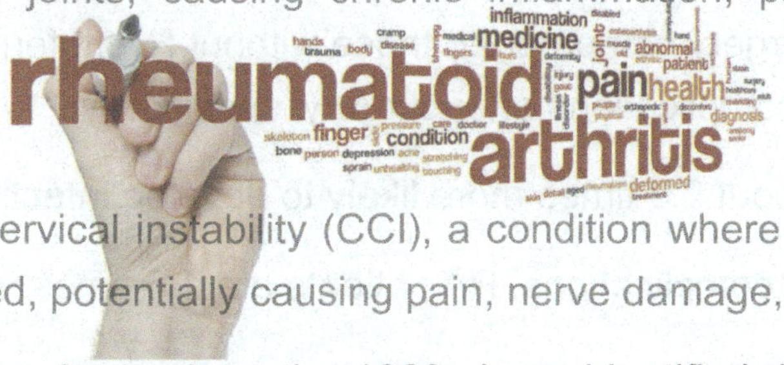

RA can lead to craniocervical instability (CCI), a condition where the bones in the upper neck become misaligned, potentially causing pain, nerve damage, or even paralysis.

Several studies dating as far back as the 1960s have identified risk factors that increase the likelihood of developing CCI in RA patients.

- Patients who have used glucocorticoids (steroids) for more than a year are at a significantly higher risk of CCI. This is because steroids can weaken bones and ligaments, making the neck more vulnerable to misalignment.
- The longer someone has RA, the greater the risk of CCI. Prolonged disease duration can result in more severe joint damage and increased inflammation in the cervical spine.
- Damage to peripheral joints, such as those in the hands or feet, is linked to an increased risk of CCI, suggesting that widespread joint involvement in RA can also affect the upper cervical spine.
- Patients who experience disability early in the course of RA are more likely to develop CCI, possibly due to more aggressive disease activity affecting the upper cervical spine.

Regular monitoring and imaging studies, such as X-rays or MRIs, can help identify early signs of instability. Early intervention, including physical therapy or surgical options like craniocervical fusion, may be necessary to prevent neurological complications.

In cases where cervical instability leads to significant pain or neurological symptoms, surgical intervention may be required. Procedures such as CCF have shown positive outcomes in RA patients, with most achieving solid fusion and improvement in symptoms. However, patients on high-dose steroids or certain medications may experience less favorable outcomes.

Rheumatoid Arthritis Patients Face Higher Risk of Surgery Complications

A study reviewed the outcomes of patients with rheumatoid arthritis (RA) undergoing craniocervical fusion surgery compared to those without RA. It found that RA patients face higher risks of several complications after surgery, specifically:

- RA patients are about 2.3 times more likely to develop infections.
- In terms of overall complications, RA patients are 1.6 times more likely to experience them.
- The risk of implant-related problems is also 3.9 times more likely in RA patients.
- RA patients are 2.45 times more likely to need re-operation after surgery.
- One other significant finding from the study is that RA patients tend to stay in the hospital longer after surgery. On average, their hospital stay is 4.6 days longer than that of non-RA patients.

This study suggested that CCF surgery for RA patients carries a higher risk of complications like infections, implant issues, and the need for re-operation. RA patients also tend to stay in the hospital longer.

It highlights the importance of closely managing RA patients' medications such as medications that suppress the immune system, and weaken the bones (osteoporosis) and health, both before and after surgery, to minimize these risks.

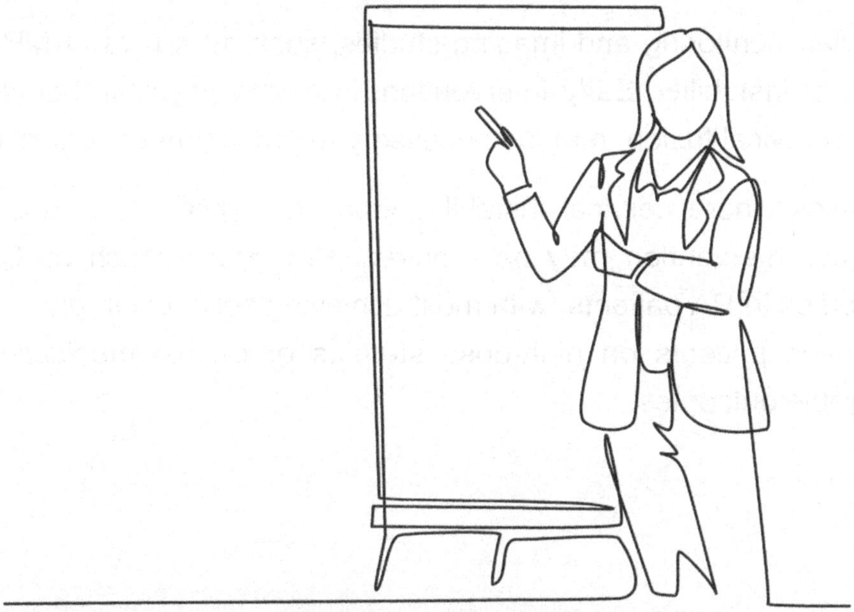

Grisel's Syndrome - "A Child's Diagnosis"

Grisel's syndrome is a serious condition that mainly affects children up to the age of 21, especially those between the ages of 2.5 and 12. It happens when the bones at the top of the spine (specifically between the first two vertebrae, called the atlas and axis) become unstable and *twisted* out of place. What makes this unusual is that it can happen *without* any trauma, like a fall or injury. Instead, it's often linked to infections in the head and neck or common ear, nose and throat (ENT) surgeries such as tonsillectomy (removal of the tonsils) or adenoidectomy (removal of the adenoids).

A 2024 review of 20 studies looked at 24 pediatric cases of Grisel's syndrome, and most of the children had recently had ENT surgeries. The symptoms appeared a few days to a few weeks after the procedures. Both boys and girls were equally affected. The best way to diagnose this condition is through a CT scan, which gives a clear, detailed picture of the bones in the neck. MRIs are also used, especially when doctors want to check for any damage to the nerves or brainstem.

Treatment depends on how severe the case is. In many cases, children get better with non-surgical treatments. These include rest, pain medications, anti-inflammatory drugs, antibiotics, and wearing a neck brace to hold the head in a stable position. However, if the condition is caught too late or is very severe, surgery may be needed to fix the bones and prevent further complications.

One of the main problems with Grisel's syndrome is that it's easy to miss. Neck pain, sore throat, or stiffness are all common after ENT procedures, so both doctors and parents may not realize something is wrong until the symptoms get worse. That's why early detection is so important. If the condition is recognized and treated early, most children recover fully and avoid long-term damage.

The studies also found more unusual symptoms such as difficulty opening the mouth, hearing loss, or a crooked face. This makes it even more important for doctors to consider Grisel's syndrome when a child complains of neck pain after surgery or an upper respiratory infection.

In short, Grisel's syndrome is rare but serious. The key to preventing complications is awareness, early diagnosis, and the right treatment. With careful attention, children with this condition can recover well and avoid long-term problems.

Grisel's Syndrome - Not Just For Kids?

Grisel's syndrome is a rare condition characterized by non-traumatic atlantoaxial subluxation (misalignment of the top two neck vertebrae) following an infection or inflammation in the head or neck area. Traditionally, this syndrome is considered a pediatric condition, often associated with upper respiratory infections or post-surgical complications. However, recent adult case reports challenge this view, indicating that Grisel's syndrome can also affect adults, albeit less frequently.

The following cases underscore the importance of recognizing that adenoid surgery and bacterial, upper respiratory, ear, throat, and other infections, may lead to CCI in adults, not just children.

Early diagnosis and appropriate treatment are crucial to prevent progression and potential neurological complications. While Grisel's syndrome remains rare in adults, the increasing number of reported cases highlights the need for heightened awareness among healthcare providers when evaluating adults with neck pain and a history of head or neck infections. More research is needed to further understand this condition.

Studies: Infections, Inflammation and Cervical Instability

Case reports have shed light on the role of infections and inflammation in the head and neck areas as a cause of CCI or cervical spine instability, emphasizing the importance of early diagnosis and appropriate treatment.

1. **Tuberculosis (TB):** A study by Sadek et al. (2011) highlighted a case where TB, caused by the bacteria Mycobacterium tuberculosis, affected the cervical spine. TB in the neck can weaken bones and put pressure on nerves, leading to pain and difficulty moving the neck. Early treatment with antibiotics is crucial to prevent long-term damage.

2. **Pyogenic Infections:** Konbaz et al. (2021) reported a case where a pyogenic (pus-forming) bacterial infection weakened the bones in the neck, causing cervical instability and pain. The patient was treated with surgery to remove infected tissue and stabilize the spine, leading to improved neck stability.

3. **Osteomyelitis caused by Staph infection:** Wang et al. (2018) reviewed data from 239 patients across 24 different studies who were treated for cervical spine osteomyelitis, a serious neck bone infection typically caused by bacteria, most

commonly Staphylococcus aureus (staph infection). The researchers found that surgical fusion was an effective treatment. Most patients experienced less pain and improved neck stability after the procedure.

4. **Upper Respiratory Infections:** In a 2003 study, Ugur et al. reported two adult cases of atlantoaxial subluxation, a condition where the top two neck vertebrae are misaligned, following upper respiratory tract infections. Both patients developed atlantoaxial instability after infections in the head or neck region. One required surgical stabilization (atlantoaxial fusion). This study challenges the traditional view that such infections primarily affect children, highlighting the need for awareness in adults as well.

5. **Upper Respiratory Infection:** Nakai et al. (2024) described a 77-year-old woman who experienced neck and shoulder pain following an upper respiratory infection. Imaging tests revealed misalignment and damage in the atlantoaxial joints (the top two neck vertebrae), causing pressure on the spinal cord. She was treated with antibiotics and a neck collar, leading to improvement over six months.

6. **Strep Throat Infection:** Ferdinandov et al. (2021) reported a 48-year-old man who developed neck pain after a streptococcal throat infection. Despite initial antibiotic treatment, his symptoms progressed, leading to CCI and neurological issues. He required surgical decompression and fusion, resulting in a full recovery.

7. **Heart Lining, Molar Extraction and Middle Ear Infections:** Kerolus et al. (2015) reported two adult cases of atlantoaxial instability (a condition where the top two neck vertebrae misaligned). One case followed endocarditis (an infection of the heart lining), while the other developed after a molar extraction and otitis media (middle ear infection). Both patients needed atlantoaxial fusion surgery to stabilize the neck, emphasizing the importance of early treatment for this condition.

8. **Back of Nose and Throat Bacterial Infection:** Chua et al. (2019) reported a 67-year-old man who developed neck pain and limited movement after surgery for nasopharyngeal cancer. Blood cultures identified the bacteria Morganella morganii as the cause of the infection. He was treated with antibiotics and a neck collar, showing significant improvement over 15 months.

9. **Adenoid Surgery:** Bocciolini et al. (2005) documented a case of Grisel's syndrome (i.e., AAI) following an adenoidectomy (surgical removal of the adenoids due to problems such as frequent infections, breathing difficulties, or ear problems). The

patient experienced persistent neck pain and stiffness after surgery, which improved with antibiotic treatment and a neck collar.

10. **COVID-19:** Barker et al. (2022) reported an 86-year-old man who developed neck pain and stiffness after a mild case of COVID-19. Imaging tests revealed misalignment of the top two neck vertebrae (AAI). He was treated with a neck collar and physical therapy, leading to significant improvement.

These medical case studies help us better understand how certain infections and surgeries may lead to CCI, causing pain, stiffness, or even nerve problems. Infections like tuberculosis (TB), strep throat, and pyogenic bacterial infections (such as staph and strep), as well as complications after surgeries like adenoidectomy or nasopharyngectomy, have been linked to some cases of CCI. While these cases show how serious the condition can become, especially when not treated early, it's important to remember that most are individual reports. More research is needed to fully understand how often these issues occur and how best to treat them.

Then and Now: Recent Trends in Diagnosis and Treatments

A study by Alan N. Cohen et al. (2017) identified the 50 most-cited articles on craniocervical junction surgery published between 1900 and 2015. These articles predominantly focused on traumatic and congenital cases, diagnostic evaluations and surgical techniques, with a notable emphasis on posterior approaches such as atlantoaxial and occipitocervical fusion. The majority of these studies were case series based on doctors' reports about one or more patients, but they were not part of a big, carefully controlled study, which underscores the need for higher-quality research in this complex field.

In contrast, recent trends in craniocervical fusion research (2016–2025) have shifted toward addressing specific patient populations and refining surgical techniques. Studies have increasingly focused on conditions like EDS and their association with CCI, leading to more targeted publications. Additionally, concerns such as postoperative dysphagia remain prevalent, prompting ongoing research into risk factors and management strategies.

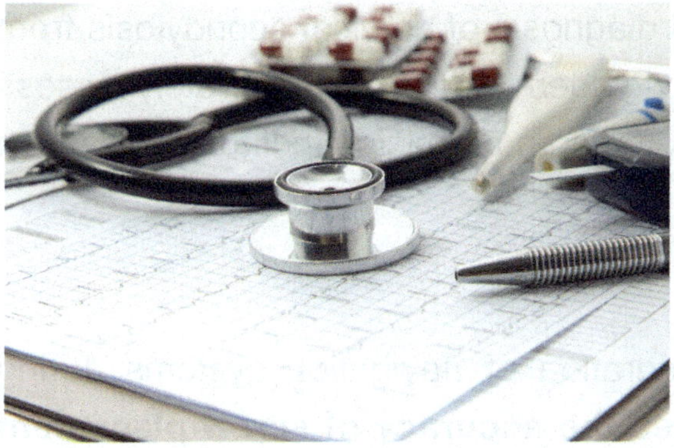

Advancements in surgical techniques, including the use of intraoperative navigation systems and 3D-printed prostheses, have been explored to enhance the safety and efficacy of craniocervical fusion procedures.

Biomechanical analyses have also been conducted to evaluate various fusion constructs, aiming to improve surgical outcomes.

Comparing these two periods reveals a shift from generalized surgical approaches to more specialized and technically advanced strategies in craniocervical fusion research. While the earlier studies laid the foundation for surgical interventions, recent research emphasizes precision, patient-specific considerations, and technological innovations to improve outcomes in CCF surgeries.

Between 2016 and 2025, diagnostic and treatment techniques for cervical spine and other disorders have evolved significantly, integrating advanced imaging modalities, artificial intelligence (AI), and innovative technologies to enhance precision and patient outcomes.

1. **Advanced Imaging Modalities**

- Dynamic CT Imaging: High-resolution dynamic 3D computed tomography (CT) (less than 1 mm slices) has become instrumental in assessing CCI. Studies have demonstrated its utility in detecting hidden or not easily seen (occult) craniocervical instability, and guiding surgical decisions.
- Upright Cone-Beam CT (uCBCT): Cone Beam Computed Tomography (CBCT) is a lower cost machinery with high imaging resolution, and helps identify CCI and Eagle syndrome by providing detailed 3D imaging.
- Dynamic Upright MRI: This imaging technique allows for assessment of the craniocervical junction (CCJ) under physiological load and movement, such as flexion, extension, and upright posture. It is particularly useful in detecting positional instability, cerebrospinal fluid flow obstruction, and subtle cord compression not evident in supine imaging.

2. **Artificial Intelligence in Imaging Diagnostics**

- AI-Assisted Analysis: Recent developments in AI have led to the creation of systems capable of automating the segmentation and diagnosis of cervical spondylosis from MRI scans. These systems utilize pathology-guided models to accurately assess anatomical structures and clinical indicators, offering a promising tool for clinicians in diagnosing CCJ disorders in the future.

3. **Intraoperative Imaging and Navigation**

- Intraoperative Navigation Systems: The integration of navigation systems during craniocervical junction surgeries has enhanced **the accuracy of screw placement and overall surgical precision**. These systems provide real-time imaging, reducing the risk of complications and improving patient outcomes.
- 3D-Printed Models: The use of patient-specific 3D-printed models derived from imaging data has facilitated preoperative planning and simulation, allowing surgeons to anticipate challenges and customize surgical approaches for craniocervical fusion procedures.

4. Robotics and Minimally Invasive Techniques

- Robotic Assistance in Surgery: Robotic systems have been employed to assist in surgeries like hip and knee replacements, offering enhanced precision in complex anatomical regions. These systems aid in navigation and instrumentation, contributing to minimally invasive approaches and potentially reducing recovery times. Given their advantages, it is hoped that CCI neurosurgeons will explore the future potential of robotic technologies to optimize surgical accuracy, reduce complications, and improve patient outcomes, especially for the placement of hardware and ensuring precise alignment, optimal screw trajectories, and minimal disruption to surrounding neural and vascular structures in the craniocervical junction.

5. Endoscopic and Minimally Invasive Approaches

- Endoscopic Transnasal Approaches: Endoscopic techniques, including transnasal approaches, have been explored for accessing the craniocervical junction, particularly in cases requiring tumor resection. These minimally invasive methods aim to reduce surgical morbidity and improve recovery times.

6. Stem Cell Therapy in Spinal Fusion

- Stem cell therapy, particularly using autologous mesenchymal stromal cells (MSCs) derived from sources like bone marrow or adipose tissue, has shown promise in promoting bone healing and fusion in spinal procedures. A clinical trial demonstrated that embedding autologous MSCs in tricalcium phosphate for posterolateral spinal fusion resulted in favorable outcomes, suggesting potential benefits for enhancing fusion rates and reducing the need for revision surgeries.

7. Training and Simulation Technologies

- Mixed Reality and Virtual Reality: Advancements in mixed reality (MR) and virtual reality (VR) have been utilized for training purposes in craniocervical junction surgery. These technologies provide immersive environments for surgical simulation, enhancing the learning experience and preparation for complex procedures.

Chapter 3 Summary

This chapter provides an evidence-based overview of what research reveals about fusion surgeries. It empowers patients to understand the medical literature, ask informed questions, and place their own treatment options within the context of current scientific knowledge. It helps patients understand what medical research says about craniocervical instability (CCI) and craniocervical fusion (CCF) surgeries. It highlights both the benefits and risks, compares different fusion approaches, and reviews complication rates and outcomes across different patient groups. By presenting medical evidence in plain language, patients and caregivers can better understand the factors that influence surgical decisions and long-term results.

- Medical studies show both the potential benefits and risks of craniocervical fusion surgery.
- Different surgical approaches such as occipitocervical fusion (OCF) and atlantoaxial fusion (AAF) are compared, with key differences explained.
- Complications are discussed in detail, including general fusion risks, specific challenges with C1–C2 fusion, and reported complication rates.
- Traumatic injuries, such as atlanto-occipital and atlantoaxial dislocations, are reviewed to show why surgical stabilization may be needed in emergencies.
- Special populations are highlighted, including patients with Down syndrome, Ehlers-Danlos syndrome (EDS), hypermobile EDS (hEDS), and rheumatoid arthritis —all of whom may face unique risks and outcomes.
- The chapter explains how dysautonomia symptoms can sometimes improve after surgery, though outcomes vary depending on whether patients have EDS or other connective tissue disorders.
- Rare but important conditions such as Grisel's syndrome in children are discussed, showing how oral surgery, throat infections, or upper respiratory infections can lead to CCI.
- Research on infection and inflammation is summarized, showing how these processes themselves may cause craniocervical instability.
- A comparison of past and current medical literature helps patients see how diagnosis and treatment trends have evolved over time.

REFERENCES

Chapter 1

1. [illegible]

2. Schatz, [illegible] (2020, October 22). [illegible]

3. [illegible]

4. [illegible] (2017). [illegible]

5. Holman [illegible]

6. [illegible]

7. Henderson, [illegible]

8. [illegible]

9. Henderson, [illegible]

10. [illegible]

11. [illegible]

1[illegible]

REFERENCES

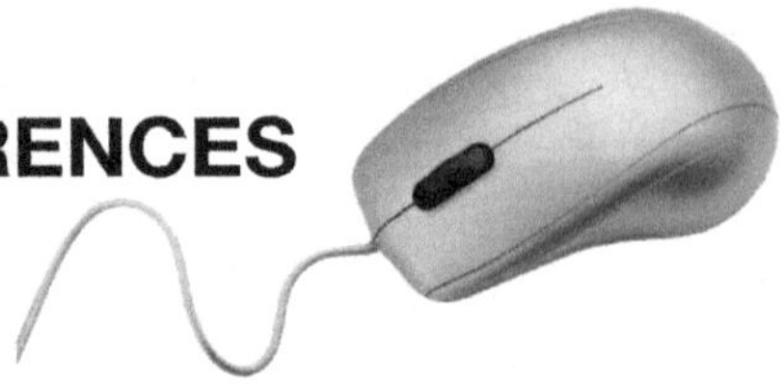

Chapter 1

1. Gilete, V. Craniocervical instability. Dr. Gilete Neurosurgery & Spine Surgery. Retrieved April 14, 2025, from https://drgilete.com/specialties-craniocervical-instability/

2. Schultz, J. R. (2020, October 12). Craniocervical instability symptoms – The 7 you need to know! Centeno-Schultz Clinic. Retrieved May 8, 2025, from https://centenoschultz.com/craniocervical-instability-symptoms/

3. Heffez DS, Ross RE, Shade-Zeldow Y, Kostas K, Shah S, Gottschalk R, Elias DA, Shepard A, Leurgans SE, Moore CG. Clinical evidence for cervical myelopathy due to Chiari malformation and spinal stenosis in a non-randomized group of patients with the diagnosis of fibromyalgia. Eur Spine J. 2004 Oct;13(6):516-23. doi: 10.1007/s00586-004-0672-x. Epub 2004 Apr 9. PMID: 15083352; PMCID: PMC3476600.

4. Heffez, D. S., Ross, R. E., Shade-Zeldow, Y., Kostas, K., Morrissey, M., Elias, D. A., & Shepard, A. (2007). Treatment of cervical myelopathy in patients with the fibromyalgia syndrome: Outcomes and implications. European Spine Journal, 16(9), 1423-1433. https://doi.org/10.1007/s00586-007-0366-2

5. Holman AJ. Positional cervical spinal cord compression and fibromyalgia: a novel comorbidity with important diagnostic and treatment implications. J Pain. 2008 Jul;9(7):613-22. doi: 10.1016/j.jpain.2008.01.339. Epub 2008 May 22. PMID: 18499527.

6. Buskila, D., Neumann, L., Vaisberg, G., Alkalay, D., & Wolfe, F. (2005). Increased rates of fibromyalgia following cervical spine injury: A controlled study of 161 cases of traumatic injury. Arthritis & Rheumatism, 53(3), 365–369. https://doi.org/10.1002/art.1780400310

7. Henderson, F. C. (2020, June 18). Ask the expert: Craniocervical instability with Dr. Fraser C. Henderson. Bobby Jones CSF. https://bobbyjonescsf.org/csf-video/henderson-ama/

8. Zhang, Y., Li, C., Dong, Q., et al. (2025). Prevalence and distribution of cervical facet joint degeneration in patients with cervical spondylotic myelopathy without/with instability and ossification of the posterior longitudinal ligament: A comparative study. European Spine Journal, 34(5), 1229–1237. https://doi.org/10.1007/s00586-025-08761-9

9. Henderson, F. C., Sr., Schubart, J. R., Narayanan, M. V., Tuchman, K., Mills, S. E., Poppe, D. J., Koby, M. B., Rowe, P. C., & Francomano, C. A. (2024). Craniocervical instability in patients with Ehlers-Danlos syndromes: Outcomes analysis following occipito-cervical fusion. Neurosurgical Review, 47(1), 27. https://doi.org/10.1007/s10143-023-02249-0

10. Bolognese, P. (2019, July 24-27). Craniocervical instability. 2019 ASAP's 31st Annual Chiari & Syringomyelia Conference. Chiari Neurosurgical Center. 2019 ASAP Conference: Craniocervical Instability, P Bolognese

11. Bolognese, P. (2020, July 22). Craniocervical Instability (CCI) [Video]. YouTube. Cranicervical Instability by Paolo Bolognese, MD Presented at the 32nd Annual Conference of the American Syringomyelia & Chiari Alliance Project, held virtually July 22–24, 2020.

12. Caring Medical Florida. (n.d.). Neck pain & cervical instability. Retrieved May 8, 2025, from https://caringmedical.com/home/conditions/neck-pain-and-cervical-instability/

13. Vij, N., Tolson, H., Kiernan, H., Agusala, V., Viswanath, O., & Urits, I. (2022, August 5). Pathoanatomy, biomechanics, and treatment of upper cervical ligamentous instability: A literature review. Orthop Rev (Pavia), 14(3), 37099. https://doi.org/10.52965/001c.37099

14. Salamon, K. S., Davies, W. H., Fuentes, M. R., Weisman, S. J., & Hainsworth, K. R. (2014). The pain frequency-severity-duration scale as a measure of pain: Preliminary validation in a pediatric chronic pain sample. Pain Research and Treatment, 2014, 653592. https://doi.org/10.1155/2014/653592 https://pubmed.ncbi.nlm.nih.gov/24579046/

15. EBSCO. (n.d.). Likert scale. EBSCO Research Starters. Retrieved May 8, 2025, from https://www.ebsco.com/research-starters/psychology/likert-scale

16. Henderson, F. C., Francomano, C. A., Koby, M., Tuchman, K., Adcock, J., & Patel, S. (2018, December 10). Cervical medullary syndrome secondary to craniocervical instability and ventral brainstem compression in hereditary hypermobility connective tissue disorders: 5-year follow-up after craniocervical reduction, fusion, and stabilization. Neurosurgical Review. https://doi.org/10.1007/s10143-018-01070-4

17. Rubin, M. (2024, March). Craniocervical junction abnormalities. Merck Manual Prof. Edition. https://www.merckmanuals.com/professional/neurologic-disorders/craniocervical-junction-abnormalities/craniocervical-junction-abnormalities. Retrieved April 14, 2005.

18. Németh, G. (2006). Health related quality of life outcome instruments. European Spine Journal, 15(Suppl 1), S44–S51. https://doi.org/10.1007/s00586-005-1046-8

19. Alentado, V. J., Lubelski, D., Steinmetz, M. P., Benzel, E. C., & Mroz, T. E. (2014). Optimal duration of conservative management prior to surgery for cervical and lumbar radiculopathy: A literature review. Global Spine Journal, 4(4), 279–286. https://doi.org/10.1055/s-0034-1387807

20. Kim, H. J., Nemani, V. M., Piyaskulkaew, C., Vargas, S. R., & Riew, K. D. (2016). Cervical radiculopathy: Incidence and treatment of 1,420 consecutive cases. Asian Spine Journal, 10(2), 231–237. https://doi.org/10.4184/asj.2016.10.2.231

21. Tarazona, D., Boody, B., Hilibrand, A. S., Stull, J., Bell, K., Fang, T., Goyal, D., Galetta, M., Kaye, D., Kepler, C. K., Kurd, M. F., Woods, B. I., Radcliff, K. E., Rihn, J. A., Anderson, D. G., Vaccaro, A. R., & Schroeder, G. D. (2019). Longer preoperative duration of symptoms negatively affects health-related quality of life after surgery for cervical radiculopathy. Spine (Phila Pa 1976), 44(10), 685–690. https://doi.org/10.1097/BRS.0000000000002924

22. Badr, H., Sobrero, M., Chen, J., Kotz, T., Genden, E., Sikora, A. G., & Miles, B. (2019). Associations between pre-, post-, and peri-operative variables and health resource use following surgery for head and neck cancer. Oral Oncology, 90, 102–108. https://doi.org/10.1016/j.oraloncology.2019.02.004

23. Narain, A. S., Hijji, F. Y., Haws, B. E., Kudaravalli, K. T., Yom, K. H., Markowitz, J., & Singh, K. (2018). Impact of body mass index on surgical outcomes, narcotics consumption, and hospital costs following anterior cervical discectomy and fusion. Journal of Neurosurgery: Spine, 28(2), 160–166. https://doi.org/10.3171/2017.6.SPINE17288

24. Jalisi, S., Jamal, B. T., & Grillone, G. A. (2017). Surgical management of long-standing Eagle syndrome. Annals of Maxillofacial Surgery, 7(2), 232–236. https://doi.org/10.4103/ams.ams_53_17

25. Ho, S., Luginbuhl, A., Finden, S., Curry, J. M., & Cognetti, D. M. (2015). Styloid/C1 transverse process juxtaposition as a cause of Eagle syndrome. Head & Neck, 37(11), E153–E156. https://doi.org/10.1002/hed.24024

26. Kumar, D., Pratap, B., Boora, N., Kumar, R., & Sah, N. K. (2021). A comparative study of medical imaging modalities. International Journal of Radiology Sciences, 3(1), 9–16. https://doi.org/10.33545/26649810.2021.v3.i1a.11

27. Levy, H. A., Karamian, B. A., Adams, A. J., Mao, J. Z., Canseco, J. A., Mandel, J., Gebeyehu, T. F., Harlamova, D., Bhatt, S. D., Heinle, J., Kaye, I. D., Woods, B. I., Hilibrand, A. S., Kepler, C. K., Vaccaro, A. R., & Schroeder, G. D. (2023). The impact of preoperative symptom duration on patient outcomes after posterior cervical decompression and fusion. Global Spine Journal, 13(8), 2463–2470. https://doi.org/10.1177/21925682221087735

28. Levi, A. D., Hurlbert, R. J., Anderson, P., Fehlings, M., Rampersaud, R., Massicotte, E. M., France, J. C., Le Huec, J. C., Hedlund, R., & Arnold, P. (2006). Neurologic deterioration secondary to unrecognized spinal instability following trauma: A multicenter study. Spine (Phila Pa 1976), 31(4), 451–458. https://doi.org/10.1097/01.brs.0000199927.78531.b5

29. Schmid, A. M., Raunig, D. L., & Miller, C. G. (2021). Radiologists and clinical trials: Part 1 The truth about reader disagreements. Therapeutic Innovation & Regulatory Science, 55(6), 1111–1121. https://doi.org/10.1007/s43441-021-00316-6

30. Brady, A. P. (2017). Error and discrepancy in radiology: Inevitable or avoidable? Insights into Imaging, 8(1), 171–182. https://doi.org/10.1007/s13244-016-0534-1

31. Herzog, R., Elgort, D. R., Flanders, A. E., & Moley, P. J. (2017). Variability in diagnostic error rates of 10 MRI centers performing lumbar spine MRI examinations on the same patient within a 3-week period. The Spine Journal, 17(4), 554–561. https://doi.org/10.1016/j.spinee.2016.11.015

32. Canadian Institute for Health Information. (2008). Medical imaging in Canada, 2007 (ISBN 978-1-55465-174-0). Ottawa, ON: Author. Retrieved from https://publications.gc.ca/collections/collection_2008/cihi-icis/H118-13-2007E.pdf

33. Jayaraman, M. V., Boxerman, J. L., Davis, L. M., Haas, R. A., & Rogg, J. M. (2012). Incidence of extrinsic compression of the internal jugular vein in unselected patients undergoing CT angiography. American Journal of Neuroradiology, 33(7), 1247–1250. https://doi.org/10.3174/ajnr.A2953

34. Farina R, Foti PV, Pennisi I, Conti A, Meli GA, Vasile T, Gozzo C, Tallamona E, Inì C, Palmucci S, Venturini M, Basile A. Stylo-Jugular Venous Compression Syndrome: Lessons Based on a Case Report. Am J Case Rep. 2021 Aug 24;22:e932035. doi: 10.12659/AJCR.932035. PMID: 34428194; PMCID: PMC8404167. https://pubmed.ncbi.nlm.nih.gov/34428194/

35. Finsterer J, Grisold W. Disorders of the lower cranial nerves. J Neurosci Rural Pract. 2015 Jul-Sep;6(3):377-91. doi: 10.4103/0976-3147.158768. PMID: 26167022; PMCID: PMC4481793. https://pubmed.ncbi.nlm.nih.gov/26167022/

36. Scerrati, A., Norri, N., Mongardi, L., Dones, F., Ricciardi, L., Trevisi, G., Menegatti, E., Zamboni, P., Cavallo, M. A., & De Bonis, P. (2021). Styloidogenic-cervical spondylotic internal jugular venous compression, a vascular disease related to several clinical neurological manifestations: Diagnosis and treatment—a comprehensive literature review. Annals of Translational Medicine, 9(8), 718. https://doi.org/10.21037/atm-20-7698

37. Bragée, B., Michos, A., Drum, B., Fahlgren, M., Szulkin, R., & Bertilson, B. C. (2020). Signs of intracranial hypertension, hypermobility, and craniocervical obstructions in patients with myalgic encephalomyelitis/chronic fatigue syndrome. Frontiers in Neurology, 11, 828. https://doi.org/10.3389/fneur.2020.00828

38. Hacking, C., Ismail, M. A. I. B., Thibodeau, R., & Radiopaedia.org. (2024, October 27). Atlantodental interval. Radiopaedia.org. https://doi.org/10.53347/rID-40483 https://radiopaedia.org/articles/atlantodental-interval

39. Martinez-Del-Campo E, Kalb S, Soriano-Baron H, Turner JD, Neal MT, Uschold T, Theodore N. Computed tomography parameters for atlantooccipital dislocation in adult patients: the occipital condyle-C1 interval. J Neurosurg Spine. 2016 Apr;24(4):535-45 doi:10.3171/2015.6.SPINE15226. Epub 2015 Dec 18. PMID: 26682597.

40. Taghva, A. (2025, June 2). 3 warning signs that show it's time to see a neurosurgeon. Alexander Taghva, MD. Retrieved June 2, 2025, from https://alextaghvamd.com/blog/3-warning-signs-show-time-see-neurosurgeon

41. Brain and Spine Neuroscience Institute. (n.d.). When it may be recommended to see a neurosurgeon. Retrieved June 2, 2025, from https://www.brainandspineni.com/blog/when-it-may-be-recommended-to-see-a-neurosurgeon/

42. Flanagan, M. F. (2015). The role of the craniocervical junction in craniospinal hydrodynamics and neurodegenerative conditions. Neurology Research International, 2015, 794829. https://doi.org/10.1155/2015/794829

43. Qureshi, A. I., Saleem, M. A., Naveed, O., Qureshi, M. A., & Wallery, S. S. (2017). Upright catheter-based cerebral angiography. Journal of Vascular and Interventional Neurology, 9(6), 14–19. https://doi.org/10.2176/jvin.9.14

44. Tubbs, R. S., Hallock, J. D., Radcliff, V., Naftel, R. P., Mortazavi, M., Shoja, M. M., Loukas, M., & Cohen-Gadol, A. A. (2011). Ligaments of the craniocervical junction: A review. Journal of Neurosurgery: Spine, 14(6), 697–709. https://doi.org/10.3171/2011.1.SPINE10612

45. Powers, B., Miller, M. D., Kramer, R. S., Martinez, S., & Gehweiler, J. A., Jr. (1979). Traumatic anterior atlanto-occipital dislocation. Neurosurgery, 4(1), 12–17. https://doi.org/10.1227/00006123-197901000-00004

46. Woo HG, Ryu J, Kim EJ, Lee KM. Styloidogenic jugular venous compression syndrome as a source of cerebral venous sinus thrombosis. Quant Imaging Med Surg. 2022 Aug;12(8):4316-4319. doi: 10.21037/qims-22-106. PMID: 35919052; PMCID: PMC9338375.

47. Farina R, Foti PV, Pennisi I, Conti A, Meli GA, Vasile T, Gozzo C, Tallamona E, Inì C, Palmucci S, Venturini M, Basile A. Stylo-Jugular Venous Compression Syndrome: Lessons Based on a Case Report. Am J Case Rep. 2021 Aug 24;22:e932035. doi: 10.12659/AJCR.932035. PMID: 34428194; PMCID: PMC8404167

48. Li, M., Sun, Y., Chan, C.C. et al. Internal jugular vein stenosis associated with elongated styloid process: five case reports and literature review. BMC Neurol **19**, 112 (2019). https://bmcneurol.biomedcentral.com/articles/10.1186/s12883-019-1344-0

49. Kosar, M. I., Atalar, M. H., Sabanclogullari, V., Tetiker, H., Erdil, F. H., Cimen, M., & Otag, I. (2011). Evaluation of the length and angulation of the styloid process in the patient with pre-diagnosis of Eagle syndrome. Folia Morphologica, 70(4), 295–299.

50. Mantovani, G., Zangrossi, P., Flacco, M. E., Di Domenico, G., Nastro Siniscalchi, E., De Ponte, F. S., Maugeri, R., De Bonis, P., Cavallo, M. A., Zamboni, P., & Scerrati, A. (2023). Styloid jugular nutcracker: The possible role of the styloid process spatial orientation—a preliminary morphometric computed study. Diagnostics, 13(2), 298. https://doi.org/10.3390/diagnostics13020298

51. Garrett, M., Consiglieri, G., Kakarla, U. K., Chang, S. W., & Dickman, C. A. (2010). Occipitoatlantal.Dislocation.Neurosurgery,66(3),A48–A55. https://doi.org/10.1227/01.NEU.0000365802.02410.C5

52. Guo, G.-M., Li, J., Diao, Q.-X., Zhu, T.-H., Song, Z.-X., Guo, Y.-Y., & Gao, Y.-Z. (2018). Cervical lordosis in asymptomatic individuals: A meta-analysis. Journal of Orthopaedic Surgery and Research, 13, 147. https://doi.org/10.1186/s13018-018-0854-6

53. Henderson, F. C. (2016). Cranio-cervical instability in patients with hypermobility connective disorders. J Spine, 5(2), 299. https://doi.org/10.4172/2165-7939.1000299

54. Nicholson, L. L., Rao, P. J., Lee, M., Wong, T. M., Cheng, R. H. Y., & Chan, C. (2023). Reference values of four measures of craniocervical stability using upright dynamic magnetic resonance imaging. La Radiologia Medica, 128(2), 330–339. https://doi.org/10.1007/s11547-023-01588-8

55. DeNunzio, G., Evans, T., Beebe, M. E., Browning, J., & Koivisto, J. (2022). Craniocervical junction visualization and radiation dose consideration utilizing cone beam computed tomography for upper cervical chiropractic clinical application: A literature review. Dose-Response, 20(2), 15593258221107515. https://doi.org/10.1177/15593258221107515

56. Mano, T., Tatsumi, S., Fujimura, S., Hotta, N., & Kido, A. (2022). Isolated bilateral hypoglossal nerve paralysis following an atlanto-occipital dislocation: A case report. Frontiers in Neurology, 13, 965717. https://doi.org/10.3389/fneur.2022.965717

57. Fisher, C. G., Sun, J. C. L., & Dvorak, M. (2001). Recognition and management of atlanto-occipital dislocation: Improving survival from an often fatal condition. Canadian Journal of Surgery, 44(6), 412–420. https://www.canjsurg.ca/content/44/6/412

58. Jorquera Moya, M., Merino Menéndez, S., Porta Etessam, J., Escribano Vera, J., & Yus Fuertes, M. (2019). Cranial nerve disorders: Clinical manifestations and topography. Radiología (English Edition), 61(2), 99-123. https://doi.org/10.1016/j.rx.2018.09.005

59. Joshi, R., & Poojary, N. (2022). The effect of muscle energy technique and posture correction exercises on pain and function in patients with non-specific chronic neck pain having forward head posture: A randomized controlled trial. International Journal of Therapeutic Massage and Bodywork, 15(2), 14-21. https://doi.org/10.3822/ijtmb.v15i2.673

60. Narain, A. S., Hijji, F. Y., Haws, B. E., Kudaravalli, K. T., Yom, K. H., Markowitz, J., & Singh, K. (2017). Impact of body mass index on surgical outcomes, narcotics consumption, and hospital costs following anterior cervical discectomy and fusion. Journal of Neurosurgery: Spine, 28(2), 160–166. https://doi.org/10.3171/2017.6.SPINE17288

61. Eubanks, J. D., Thorpe, S. W., Cheruvu, V. K., Braly, B. A., & Kang, J. D. (2010). Does smoking influence fusion rates in posterior cervical arthrodesis with lateral mass instrumentation? Clinical Orthopaedics and Related Research, 469(3), 696–701. https://doi.org/10.1007/s11999-010-1575-2

62. Zileli, M., & Akıntürk, N. (2022). Complications of occipitocervical fixation: Retrospective review of 128 patients with 5-year mean follow-up. European Spine Journal, 31(2), 311–326. https://doi.org/10.1007/s00586-021-07037-2

63. Quinn, T. J., Dawson, J., Walters, M. R., & Lees, K. R. (2009). Exploring the reliability of the Modified Rankin Scale. Stroke, 40(3), 758–763. https://doi.org/10.1161/STROKEAHA.108.522516

64. Nasreddine, Z. S., Phillips, N. A., Bédirian, V., Charbonneau, S., Whitehead, V., Collin, I., Cummings, J. L., & Chertkow, H. (2005). The Montreal Cognitive Assessment, MoCA: A brief screening tool for mild cognitive impairment. Journal of the American Geriatrics Society, 53(4), 695–699. https://doi.org/10.1111/j.1532-5415.2005.53221.x

65. National Institute of Neurological Disorders and Stroke [NIHNINDS]. (2024, January 5). ME/CFS Research Roadmap Webinar – Lesser Studied Pathologies [Video]. YouTube. https://youtu.be/A-RN1yjwtIs?si=fiTpEo41fVazzu8S

66. Henderson, F. C., Sr., Henderson, F. C., Jr., Wilson, W. A., 4th, Mark, A. S., & Koby, M. (2018). Utility of the clivo-axial angle in assessing brainstem deformity: Pilot study and literature review. Neurosurgical Review, 41(1), 149–163. https://doi.org/10.1007/s10143-017-0830-3

67. Sayah, A., Farley, A. D., Munoz, E. C., Sandhu, F. A., & Berkowitz, F. (2021). Normal range of clivoaxial angle in adults using flexion and extension cervical magnetic resonance imaging scans. Neuroradiology Journal, 34(4), 348–354. https://doi.org/10.1177/1971400921998982

68. Tam, S. K. P., Chia, J., Brodbelt, A., & Foroughi, M. (2021). Assessment of patients with a Chiari malformation type I. Brain Spine, 2, 100850. https://doi.org/10.1016/j.bas.2021.100850

69. Jayaraman, M. V., Boxerman, J. L., Davis, L. M., Haas, R. A., & Rogg, J. M. (2012). Incidence of extrinsic compression of the internal jugular vein in unselected patients undergoing CT angiography. American Journal of Neuroradiology, 33(7), 1247–1250. https://doi.org/10.3174/ajnr.A2953

70. Scerrati, A., Norri, N., Mongardi, L., Dones, F., Ricciardi, L., Trevisi, G., Menegatti, E., Zamboni, P., Cavallo, M. A., & De Bonis, P. (2021). Styloidogenic-cervical spondylotic internal jugular venous compression, a vascular disease related to several clinical neurological manifestations: Diagnosis and treatment—a comprehensive literature review. Annals of Translational Medicine, 9(8), 718. https://doi.org/10.21037/atm-20-7698

71. Bragée, B., Michos, A., Drum, B., Fahlgren, M., Szulkin, R., & Bertilson, B. C. (2020). Signs of intracranial hypertension, hypermobility, and craniocervical obstructions in patients with myalgic encephalomyelitis/chronic fatigue syndrome. Frontiers in Neurology, 11, 828. https://doi.org/10.3389/fneur.2020.00828

72. Flanagan, M. F. (2015). The role of the craniocervical junction in craniospinal hydrodynamics and neurodegenerative conditions. Neurology Research International, 2015, 794829. https://doi.org/10.1155/2015/794829

73. Qureshi, A. I., Saleem, M. A., Naveed, O., Qureshi, M. A., & Wallery, S. S. (2017). Upright catheter-based cerebral angiography. Journal of Vascular and Interventional Neurology, 9(6), 14–19. https://doi.org/10.2176/jvin.9.14

74. Alentado, V. J., Lubelski, D., Steinmetz, M. P., Benzel, E. C., & Mroz, T. E. (2014). Optimal duration of conservative management prior to surgery for cervical and lumbar radiculopathy: A literature review. Global Spine Journal, 4(4), 279–286. https://doi.org/10.1055/s-0034-1387807 SAGE Journals

75. Kim, H. J., Nemani, V. M., Piyaskulkaew, C., Vargas, S. R., & Riew, K. D. (2016). Cervical radiculopathy: Incidence and treatment of 1,420 consecutive cases. Asian Spine Journal, 10(2), 231–237. https://doi.org/10.4184/asj.2016.10.2.231

76. Tarazona, D., Boody, B., Hilibrand, A. S., Stull, J., Bell, K., Fang, T., Goyal, D., Galetta, M., Kaye, D., Kepler, C. K., Kurd, M. F., Woods, B. I., Radcliff, K. E., Rihn, J. A., Anderson, D. G., Vaccaro, A. R., & Schroeder, G. D. (2019). Longer preoperative duration of symptoms negatively affects health-related quality of life after surgery for cervical radiculopathy. Spine (Phila Pa 1976), 44(10), 685–690. https://doi.org/10.1097/BRS.0000000000002924

77. Held, M. E., Farsi, S., Creighton, E. R. W., Davis, K. P., King, D. L., & Suen, J. Y. (2024). Eagle syndrome presentation and outcomes in a large surgical case series. Laryngoscope Investigative Otolaryngology, 9(4), e1289. https://doi.org/10.1002/lio2.1289

78. Badr, H., Sobrero, M., Chen, J., Kotz, T., Genden, E., Sikora, A. G., & Miles, B. (2019). Associations between pre-, post-, and peri-operative variables and health resource use following surgery for head and neck cancer. Oral Oncology, 90, 102–108. https://doi.org/10.1016/j.oraloncology.2019.02.004

79. Jalisi, M., Jamal, B. T., & Grillone, G. A. (2017). Surgical management of long-standing Eagle syndrome. Annals of Maxillofacial Surgery, 7(2), 232–236. https://doi.org/10.4103/ams.ams_53_17

80. Levy, H. A., Karamian, B. A., Adams, A. J., Mao, J. Z., Canseco, J. A., Mandel, J., Gebeyehu, T. F., Harlamova, D., Bhatt, S. D., Heinle, J., Kaye, I. D., Woods, B. I., Hilibrand, A. S., Kepler, C. K., Vaccaro, A. R., & Schroeder, G. D. (2023). The impact of preoperative symptom duration on patient outcomes after posterior cervical decompression and fusion. Global Spine Journal, 13(8), 2463–2470. https://doi.org/10.1177/21925682221087735

81. Henderson, F. C., Francomano, C. A., Koby, M., Tuchman, K., Adcock, J., Patel, S., & others. (2019). Cervical medullary syndrome secondary to craniocervical instability and ventral brainstem compression in hereditary hypermobility connective tissue disorders: 5-year follow-up after craniocervical reduction, fusion, and stabilization. Neurosurgical Review, 42(4), 915–936. https://doi.org/10.1007/s10143-018-01070-4

82. Henderson, F. C., Sr., Schubart, J. R., Narayanan, M. V., Tuchman, K., Koby, M. B., Rowe, P. C., & Francomano, C. A. (2024). Craniocervical instability in patients with Ehlers-Danlos syndromes: Outcomes analysis following occipito-cervical fusion. Neurosurgical Review, 47(1), 27. https://doi.org/10.1007/s10143-023-02249-0

83. Machida, M., Rocos, B., Taira, K., Nemoto, N., Oikawa, N., Kinoshita, T., Kozu, T., & Nakanishi, K. (2022). The association between radiographic and MRI cervical spine parameters in patients with Down syndrome. Cureus, 14(5), e25046. https://doi.org/10.7759/cureus.25046

84. Chen, Y., Zhuang, Z., Qi, W., Yang, H., Chen, Z., Wang, X., & Kong, K. (2011). A three-dimensional study of the atlantodental interval in a normal Chinese population using reformatted computed tomography. Surgical and Radiologic Anatomy, 33(11), 801-806. https://doi.org/10.1007/s00276-011-0891-2

85. Rojas, C. A., Bertozzi, J. C., Martinez, C. R., & Whitlow, J. (2007). Reassessment of the craniocervical junction: Normal values on CT. AJNR American Journal of Neuroradiology, 28(9), 1819–1823. https://doi.org/10.3174/ajnr.A0660

86. Normal range of clivoaxial angle in adults using flexion and extension cervical magnetic resonance imaging scans. (2021). Journal of Neurosurgery: Spine, 35(2), 183–188. https://doi.org/10.3171/2021.2.SPINE201053

87. Yang, S. Y., Boniello, A. J., Poorman, C. E., Chang, A. L., Wang, S., & Passias, P. G. (2014). A review of the diagnosis and treatment of atlantoaxial dislocations. Global Spine Journal, 4(3), 197-210. https://doi.org/10.1055/s-0034-1378257

88. Wang, C., Yan, M., Zhou, H., Wang, S., & Dang, G. (2007). Atlantoaxial transarticular screw fixation with morselized autograft and without additional internal fixation: Technical description and report of 57 cases. Spine, 32(6), 643-646. https://doi.org/10.1097/01.brs.0000255823.88899.76

89. Chen, Q., Brahimaj, B. C., Khanna, R., Kerolus, M. G., Tan, L. A., David, B. T., & Fessler, R. G. (2020). Posterior atlantoaxial fusion: A comprehensive review of surgical techniques and relevant vascular anomalies. Journal of Spine Surgery, 6(1), 164-172. https://doi.org/10.21037/jss.2020.01.13

90. Elbadrawi, A. M., & Elkhateeb, T. M. (2017). Transoral approach for odontoidectomy efficacy and safety. HSS Journal®, 13(3), 276-281. https://doi.org/10.1007/s11420-017-9576-9

91. Munakomi, S., Tamrakar, K., Chaudhary, P. K., & Bhattarai, B. (2016). Anterior single odontoid screw placement for type II odontoid fractures: Our modified surgical technique and initial results in a cohort study of 15 patients. F1000 Research, 5, 1681. https://doi.org/10.12688/f1000research.9305.1

92. Michel, C., Dijanic, C., Abdelmalek, G., Sudah, S., Kerrigan, D., & Yalamanchili, P. (2022). Upper cervical spine instability systematic review: A bibliometric analysis of the 100 most influential publications. Journal of Spine Surgery, 8(2), 266-272. https://doi.org/10.21037/jss-22-18

93. Joaquim, A. F., & Appenzeller, S. (2014). Cervical spine involvement in rheumatoid arthritis—a systematic review. Autoimmunity Reviews, 13(12), 1195-1202. https://doi.org/10.1016/j.autrev.2014.09.004

94. Shah, A., Vutha, R., Prasad, A., & Goel, A. (2023). Central or axial atlantoaxial dislocation and craniovertebral junction alterations: A review of 393 patients treated over 12 years. Neurosurgical Focus, 54(3), E13. https://doi.org/10.3171/2023.1.FOCUS22243

95. Manent, L., Higuera, J. G., Lewis, K., Angulo, O., & Solano, M. E. (2022). Radiological improvements in symmetry of the lateral atlantodental interval and in C1 tilt after the application of the Atlasprofilax method: A case series. Qeios. https://doi.org/10.32388/YHSZFH

96. Woods, R. O., Inceoglu, S., Akpolat, Y. T., Cheng, W. K., Jabo, B., & Danisa, O. (2018). C1 lateral mass displacement and transverse atlantal ligament failure in Jefferson's fracture: A biomechanical study of the "Rule of Spence." Neurosurgery, 82(2), 226–231. https://doi.org/10.1093/neuros/nyx194

97. Nicholson, L. L., Rao, P. J., Lee, M., Wong, T. M., Cheng, R. H., & Chan, C. (2023). Reference values of four measures of craniocervical stability using upright dynamic magnetic resonance imaging. La Radiologia Medica, 128(3), 330-339. https://doi.org/10.1007/s11547-023-01575-0

98. Sen, R. D., Martinez, V., Eaton, J., Holdefer, R. N., & Ellenbogen, R. G. (2023). Intraoperative neuromonitoring for pediatric Chiari decompression: When is it useful? Neurosurgical Focus, 54(3), E9. https://doi.org/10.3171/2023.1.FOCUS22242

99. Lohkamp, L. N., Marathe, N., & Fehlings, M. G. (2022). Craniocervical instability in Ehlers-Danlos syndrome—A systematic review of diagnostic and surgical treatment criteria. Global Spine Journal, 12(8), 1862-1871. https://doi.org/10.1177/21925682221110416

100. Henderson, F. C., Francomano, C. A., Koby, M., Tuchman, K., Adcock, J., & Patel, S. (2019). Cervical medullary syndrome secondary to craniocervical instability and ventral brainstem compression in hereditary hypermobility connective tissue disorders: 5-year follow-up after craniocervical reduction, fusion, and stabilization. Neurosurgical Review, 42(4), 915-936. https://doi.org/10.1007/s10143-018-01070-4

101. Henderson, F. C., Rosenbaum, R., Narayanan, M., Mackall, J., & Koby, M. (2020). Optimizing alignment parameters during craniocervical stabilization and fusion: A technical note. Cureus, 12(3), e7117. https://doi.org/10.7759/cureus.7117

102. Patkar, S. V., & Patkar, P. (2021). Basilar invagination: Surgical treatment by novel anterior implant. Journal of Orthopaedic Case Reports, 11(6), 36-39. https://doi.org/10.13107/jocr.2021.v11.i06.2225

103. Bransford, R. J., Alton, T. B., Patel, A. R., & Bellabarba, C. (2014). Upper cervical spine trauma. Journal of the American Academy of Orthopaedic Surgeons, 22(11), 718-729. https://doi.org/10.5435/JAAOS-22-11-718

104. Canadian Association of Radiologists. (2018, April 26-29). CAR 2018 annual scientific meeting | Congrès scientifique annuel [Program]. Montréal, Le Centre Sheraton. https://car-asm.ca/wp-content/uploads/2024/08/CAR-2018-Program.pdf

105. Saxena, A. (2017). Upper cervical trauma. Journal of Spine & Neurosurgery, 6(5). https://doi.org/10.4172/2325-9701.1000284

106. Vijay Kumar, G., & Gomatam, R. (2022). Approach to upper cervical trauma. Indian Spine Journal, 5(1), 10-23. https://doi.org/10.4103/ISJ.ISJ_31_21

107. Kauppi, M., Leppänen, L., Heikkilä, S., Lahtinen, T., & Kautiainen, H. (1998). Active conservative treatment of atlantoaxial subluxation in rheumatoid arthritis. British Journal of Rheumatology, 37(4), 417-420. https://doi.org/10.1093/rheumatology/37.4.417

108. Bidot, S., Saindane, A. M., Peragallo, J. H., Bruce, B. B., Newman, N. J., & Biousse, V. (2015). Brain imaging in idiopathic intracranial hypertension. Journal of Neuro-Ophthalmology, 35(4), 400-411. https://doi.org/10.1097/WNO.0000000000000303

109. Bejjani, G. K. (2003). Association of the adult Chiari malformation and idiopathic intracranial hypertension: More than a coincidence. Medical Hypotheses, 60(6), 859-863. https://doi.org/10.1016/s0306-9877(03)00064-1

110. Hepworth, E. J., Love, A. V., & Hartford, R. L. (2021). Intracranial hypertension secondary to venous outflow obstruction. Journal of Neurological Surgery B: Skull Base, 82(Suppl 2), S65-S270. https://doi.org/10.1055/s-0041-1725347

111. Parkkola, R. K., Rytökoski, U. M., Komu, M. E. S., & Thomsen, C. (2000). Cerebrospinal fluid flow in the cervical spinal canal in patients with chronic neck pain. Acta Radiologica, 41(6), 578-583. https://doi.org/10.1080/028418500127345938

112. Ellingson, B. M., Woodworth, D. C., Leu, K., Salamon, N., & Holly, L. T. (2019). Spinal cord perfusion MR imaging implicates both ischemia and hypoxia in the pathogenesis of cervical spondylosis. World Neurosurgery, 128, e773-e781. https://doi.org/10.1016/j.wneu.2019.04.253

113. Flanagan, M. F. (2015). The role of the craniocervical junction in craniospinal hydrodynamics and neurodegenerative conditions. Neurological Research International, 2015, 794829. https://doi.org/10.1155/2015/794829

114. Puustinen, T., Tervonen, J., Avellan, C., Jyrkkänen, H. K., Paterno, J. J., Hartikainen, P., Vanhanen, U., Leinonen, V., Lehto, S. M., Elomaa, A. P., & Huttunen, T. J. (2019). Psychiatric disorders are a common prognostic marker for worse outcome in patients with idiopathic intracranial hypertension. Clinical Neurology and Neurosurgery, 186, 105527. https://doi.org/10.1016/j.clineuro.2019.105527

115. Xiong, L., & Wang, Z. (2023). Intracranial hypertension due to bilateral internal jugular venous occlusion in Eagle syndrome: A case report. Heliyon, 9(5), e16188. https://doi.org/10.1016/j.heliyon.2023.e16188

116. Xu, Z., Shi, P., & Zhang, P. (2024). Eagle syndrome: A rare neuropathic disorder affecting head and neck. Medicine (Baltimore), 103(19), e38128. https://doi.org/10.1097/MD.0000000000038128

117. Galletta, K., Siniscalchi, E., Cicciù, M., Velo, G., & Granata, G. (2020). Is Eagle jugular syndrome an underestimated potentially life-threatening disease? Canadian Journal of Neurological Sciences, 47(4), 581–582. https://doi.org/10.1017/cjn.2020.48

118. Goel A, Blaskovich S. Rotatory and translatory "central or axial" atlantoaxial instability - Role of dynamic imaging. J Craniovertebr Junction Spine. 2023 Oct-Dec;14(4):311-312. doi: 10.4103/jcvjs.jcvjs_163_23.. Epub 2023 Nov 29. PMID:38268686; PMCID: PMC10805153.

119. Xiong, L., & Wang, Z. (2019). Eagle syndrome as a cause of cerebral venous sinus thrombosis. Canadian Journal of Neurological Sciences, 46(3), 301-304. https://doi.org/10.1017/cjn.2019.49

120. Xu, Z., Shi, P., & Zhang, P. (2024). Eagle syndrome: A rare neuropathic disorder affecting head and neck. Medicine (Baltimore), 103(19), e38128. https://doi.org/10.1097/MD.0000000000038128

121. Neurological Phenotypes and Treatment Outcomes in Eagle Syndrome: Systematic Review and Meta-Analysis Peer J. (2023). Neurological phenotypes and treatment outcomes in Eagle syndrome: Systematic review and meta-analysis. PeerJ, 11, e17423. https://doi.org/10.7717/peerj.17423

122. Milhorat, T. H., Bolognese, P. A., Nishikawa, M., McDonnell, N. B., & Francomano, C. A. (2007). Syndrome of occipitoatlantoaxial hypermobility, cranial settling, and Chiari malformation Type I in patients with hereditary disorders of connective tissue. Journal of Neurosurgery: Spine, 7(6), 601–609. https://doi.org/10.3171/SPI-07/12/601

123. Goel, A. (2012). Instability and basilar invagination. Journal of Craniovertebral Junction and Spine, 3(1), 1-2. https://doi.org/10.4103/0974-8237.110115

124. Algattas, H. N., Alattar, A. A., Okonkwo, D. O., Wang, E. W., Snyderman, C. H., Hamilton, D. K., Friedlander, R. M., Zenonos, G. A., & Gardner, P. A. (2023). A novel classification and management scheme for craniocervical junction disorders with ventral neural element compression. Journal of Neurosurgery, 140(2), 585–594. https://doi.org/10.3171/2023.5.JNS23677

125. Henderson, F. C., Francomano, C. A., Koby, M., et al. (2019). Cervical medullary syndrome secondary to craniocervical instability and ventral brainstem compression in hereditary hypermobility connective tissue disorders: 5-year follow-up after craniocervical reduction, fusion, and stabilization. Neurosurgical Review, 42(4), 915–936. https://doi.org/10.1007/s10143-018-01070-4.

126. Goel, A., & Shah, A. (2009). Reversal of longstanding musculoskeletal changes in basilar invagination after surgical decompression and stabilization. Journal of Neurosurgery: Spine, 10(3), 220–227. https://doi.org/10.3171/2008.12.SPINE08499

127. Sheehan, S., Bauer, R. B., & Meyer, J. S. (1960). Vertebral artery compression in cervical spondylosis. Neurology, 10(11), 968–973. https://doi.org/10.1212/WNL.10.11.968

128. Henderson, F. C., Francomano, C. A., Koby, M., et al. (2019). Cervical medullary syndrome secondary to craniocervical instability and ventral brainstem compression in hereditary hypermobility connective tissue disorders: 5-year follow-up after craniocervical reduction, fusion, and stabilization. Neurosurgical Review, 42(4), 915–936. https://doi.org/10.1007/s10143-018-01070-4

129. Badhey A, Jategaonkar A, Anglin Kovacs AJ, Kadakia S, De Deyn PP, Ducic Y, Schantz S, Shin E. Eagle syndrome: A comprehensive review. Clin Neurol Neurosurg. 2017 Aug;159:34-38. doi: 10.1016/j.clineuro.2017.04.021. https://doi.org/10.1016/j.clineuro.2017.04.021

130. Halalmeh, D. R., Vrana, A., Mercer, L., & Moisi, M. (2024, January 24). Traumatic Eagle syndrome: A rare cause of neck pain and headache in trauma patients. American Journal of Case Reports, 25, e942595. https://doi.org/10.12659/AJCR.942595. PMID: 38263689; PMCID: PMC10825704.

131. Nakanishi, K., Tanaka, N., Kamei, N., Nakamae, T., Izumi, B., Ohta, R., Fujioka, Y., & Ochi, M. (2013). Use of prone position magnetic resonance imaging for detecting the terminal filum in patients with occult tethered cord syndrome. Journal of Neurosurgery: Spine, 18(1), 76–84. https://doi.org/10.3171/2012.10.SPINE12321

132. Aoun, S. G., El Ahmadieh, T. Y., Vance, A. Z., Neeley, O., & Morrill, K. C. (2019). The use of prone magnetic resonance imaging to rule out tethered cord in patients with structural spine anomalies: A diagnostic technical note for surgical decision-making. Cureus, 11(3), e4221. https://doi.org/10.7759/cureus.4221

133. Arun, A., Amans, M. R., Higgins, N., Brinjikji, W., Sattur, M., Satti, S. R., Nakaji, P., Luciano, M., Huisman, T. A., Moghekar, A., Pereira, V. M., Meng, R., Fargen, K., & Hui, F. K. (2022). A proposed framework for cerebral venous congestion. Neuroradiology Journal, 35(1), 94–111. https://doi.org/10.1177/19714009211029261

134. Fargen, K. M. (2021). Idiopathic intracranial hypertension explained: A guide for patients and families. Springer. https://doi.org/10.1007/978-3-030-80041-3

135. Ho, S., Luginbuhl, A., Finden, S., Curry, J. M., & Cognetti, D. M. (2015). Styloid/C1 transverse process juxtaposition as a cause of Eagle syndrome. Head & Neck, 37(11), E153–E156. https://doi.org/10.1002/hed.24024

136. Brassart, N., Deforche, M., Goutte, A., & Wery, D. (2020). A rare vascular complication of Eagle syndrome highlighted by CTA with neck flexion. Radiology Case Reports, 15(8), 1408–1412. https://doi.org/10.1016/j.radcr.2020.05.052

137. Bai, C., Wang, Z., Guan, J., Jin, K., Ding, Y., Ji, X., & Meng, R. (2020). Clinical characteristics and neuroimaging findings in Eagle syndrome induced internal jugular vein stenosis. Annals of Translational Medicine, 8(4), 97. https://doi.org/10.21037/atm.2019.12.93

138. Tanaka, Y., Anami, H., Kurihara, H., Miyao, S., Nakamoto, H., Kubota, Y., & Kawamata, T. (2021). Eagle syndrome with hidden stylocarotid syndrome examined using dynamic ultrasonography: Illustrative case. Journal of Neurosurgery Case Lessons, 1(26), CASE21286. https://doi.org/10.3171/CASE21286

139. Kamal, A., Nazir, R., Usman, M., Salam, B. U., & Sana, F. (2014). Eagle syndrome: Radiological evaluation and management. Journal of the Pakistan Medical Association, 64(11), 1315–1317. PMID: 25831655 https://pubmed.ncbi.nlm.nih.gov/25831655/

140. Mehta, A., Chai, E., Berglund, K., Rizzo, E., Moreno, J., & Gelfman, L. P. (2021). Using admission Karnofsky Performance Status as a guide for palliative care discharge needs. Journal of Palliative Medicine, 24(6), 910–913. https://doi.org/10.1089/jpm.2020.0543

141. Russek, L. N., Block, N. P., Byrne, E., Chalela, S., Chan, C., Comerford, M., Frost, N., Hennessey, S., McCarthy, A., Nicholson, L. L., Parry, J., Simmonds, J., Stott, P. J., Thomas, L., Treleaven, J., Wagner, W., & Hakim, A. (2023). Presentation and physical therapy management of upper cervical instability in patients with symptomatic generalized joint hypermobility: International expert consensus recommendations. Frontiers in Medicine, 9, 1072764. https://doi.org/10.3389/fmed.2022.1072764

142. Smith, A., Andruski, B., Deng, G., & Burnham, R. (2023). Cervical facet joint platelet-rich plasma in people with chronic whiplash-associated disorders: A prospective case series of longer term 6- and 12-month outcomes. Interventional Pain Medicine, 2(1), 100237. https://doi.org/10.1016/j.inpm.2023.100237

143. Stone, J. E., Campbell, C., Tabor, J. B., Bonfield, S., Machan, M., Shan, R. L. P., & Debert, C. T. (2024). Ultrasound guided platelet rich plasma injections for post-traumatic greater occipital neuralgia following concussion: A pilot randomized controlled trial. Frontiers in Neurology, 15, 1400057. https://doi.org/10.3389/fneur.2024.1400057

144. Williams, C., Jerome, M., Fausel, C., Dodson, E., Stemper, I., & Centeno, C. (2021). Regenerative injection treatments utilizing platelet products and prolotherapy for cervical spine pain: A functional spinal unit approach. Cureus, 13(10), e18608. https://doi.org/10.7759/cureus.18608

145. Kauppi, M., & Anttila, P. (1995). A stiff collar can restrict atlantoaxial instability in rheumatoid cervical spine in selected cases. Annals of the Rheumatic Diseases, 54(4), 305-307. https://doi.org/10.1136/ard.54.4.305

146. Healthline. (n.d.). Cervical collar: Types, uses, and more. Retrieved April 14, 2025, from https://www.healthline.com/health/cervical-collar

147. HealthCentral. (n.d.). When to use heat versus ice for pain. Retrieved April 14, 2025, from https://www.healthcentral.com/pain-management/when-use-heat-versus-ice-pain

148. Journal of Orthopaedic & Sports Physical Therapy. (2009). Volume 39(5), 400-417. https://doi.org/10.2519/jospt.2009.2930.

149. Biester, R. C. (2013). Outcome scales and neuropsychological outcome. In P. D. Le Roux, J. M. Levine, & W. A. Kofke (Eds.), Monitoring in neurocritical care (pp. 107–113.e2). W.B. Saunders. https://doi.org/10.1016/B978-1-4377-0167-8.00012-1

150. Herdman, M., Gudex, C., Lloyd, A., Janssen, M., Kind, P., Parkin, D., & Badia, X. (2011). Development and preliminary testing of the new five-level version of EQ-5D (EQ-5D-5L). Quality of Life Research, 20(10), 1727–1736. https://doi.org/10.1007/s11136-011-9903-x

151. Klepinowski, T., & Sagan, L. (2022). EuroQol-5 dimensions health-related quality of life questionnaire in craniovertebral instability treated with posterior fixation with or without occipital plating: A comparative study with matched datasets. Journal of Craniovertebral Junction and Spine, 13(1), 72–79. https://doi.org/10.4103/jcvjs.jcvjs_125_21

152. Eran, A., Yousem, D. M., & Izbudak, I. (2016). Asymmetry of the odontoid lateral mass interval in pediatric trauma CT: Do we need to investigate further? AJNR. American Journal of Neuroradiology, 37(1), 176-179. https://doi.org/10.3174/ajnr.A4492

153. Guenkel, S., Scheyerer, M. J., Osterhoff, G., et al. (2016). It is the lateral head tilt, not head rotation, causing an asymmetry of the odontoid-lateral mass interspace. European Journal of Trauma and Emergency Surgery, 42(6), 749–754. https://doi.org/10.1007/s00068-015-0602-0

154. Billmann, F., Bokor-Billmann, T., Burnett, C., & Kiffner, E. (2013). Occurrence and significance of odontoid lateral mass interspace asymmetry in trauma patients. World Journal of Surgery, 37(8), 1988-1995. https://doi.org/10.1007/s00268-013-2048-z

155. Zhao, X., Wu, Z. X., Han, B. J., Yan, Y. B., Zhang, Y., & Lei, W. (2013). Three-dimensional analysis of cervical spine segmental motion in rotation. Archives of Medical Science, 9(3), 515-520. https://doi.org/10.5114/aoms.2013.35325

156. Penning, L., & Wilmink, J. T. (1987). Rotation of the cervical spine: A CT study in normal subjects. Spine(Philadelphia,Pa.1976),12(8), 732-738. https://doi.org/10.1097/00007632-198710000-00003

157. Liu, K., Niu, X., Wu, C., Guo, L., Liu, C., Song, H., & Chhabra, A. (2013). Normative data on axial rotation of atlanto-occipital joint on 3 Tesla MRI using a simple and reliable method of calculation. Acta Radiologica, 54(10), 1175-1181. https://doi.org/10.1177/0284185113491253

158. Leong, N., Lim, E., & Ho, C. L. (2021). Radiological signs in traumatic cervical facet joint dislocations. Journal of the Belgian Society of Radiology, 105(1), 8. https://doi.org/10.5334/jbsr.2314

159. Kirpalani, D., & Mitra, R. (2008). Cervical facet joint dysfunction: A review. Archives of Physical Medicine and Rehabilitation, 89(4), 770-774. https://doi.org/10.1016/j.apmr.2007.11.028

160. Bhatti, A. B., & Kim, S. (2016). Application of the Harms technique to treat undiagnosed intractable C1-C2 unilateral neck pain: A case report. Cureus, 8(9), e793. https://doi.org/10.7759/cureus.793

161. Joaquim, A. F., Evangelista Santos Barcelos, A. C., Daniel, J. W., & Botelho, R. V. (2023). Chamberlain's line violation in basilar invagination patients compared with normal subjects: A systematic literature review and meta-analysis. World Neurosurgery, 173, e364-e370. https://doi.org/10.1016/j.wneu.2023.02.057

162. Guo, X., Han, Z., Xiao, J., Chen, Q., Chen, F., Guo, Q., Yang, J., & Ni, B. (2019). Cervicomedullary angle as an independent radiological predictor of postoperative neurological outcome in type A basilar invagination. Scientific Reports, 9(1), 19364. https://doi.org/10.1038/s41598-019-55780-w

163. Ebrahimzadeh, S. A., Loth, F., Ibrahimy, A., Nwotchouang, B. S. T., & Bhadelia, R. A. (2022). Diagnostic utility of parasagittal measurements of tonsillar herniation in Chiari I malformation. Neuroradiology Journal, 35(2), 233-239. https://doi.org/10.1177/19714009211041524

164. Congress of Neurological Surgeons. (n.d.). New CNS guideline for patients with Chiari malformation.CNS.Retrieved.from https://www.cns.org/about/press-room-detail/new-cns-guideline-patients-with-chiari-malformation

165. Bolognese, P. A., Brodbelt, A., Bloom, A. B., & Kula, R. W. (2019). Chiari I malformation: Opinions on diagnostic trends and controversies from a panel of 63 international experts. World Neurosurgery, 130, e9-e16. https://doi.org/10.1016/j.wneu.2019.05.098

166. Goel, A. (2014). Is atlantoaxial instability the cause of Chiari malformation? Outcome analysis of 65 patients treated by atlantoaxial fixation. Spine, 22(2), 116–127. https://doi.org/10.3171/2014.10.SPINE14176

167. Goel, A., Vutha, R., Shah, A., Ranjan, S., Jadhav, N., & Jadhav, D. (2020). Atlantoaxial fixation for failed foramen magnum decompression in patients with Chiari formation. Journal of Craniovertebral Junction & Spine, 11(3), 186-192. https://doi.org/10.4103/jcvjs.JCVJS_113_20

168.Goel, A. (2025). Chiari formation and atlantoaxial instability. Commentary on minimally invasive non-expansile tubular extradural posterior fossa decompression (MINTED technique) for the management of Chiari I.5 malformation: Historical overview of surgical techniques, technical note, proof of concept, illustrative case, and case series. Archives of Neurosurgery, 1(1), Article 10. https://doi.org/10.71119/2992-8478.1007

169.Rojas CA, Bertozzi JC, Martinez CR, Whitlow J. Reassessment of the craniocervical junction: normal values on CT. AJNR Am J Neuroradiol. 2007 Oct;28(9):1819-23. doi: 10.3174/ajnr.A0660. Epub 2007 Sep 24. PMID: 17893223; PMCID: PMC8134200.

Chapter 2

170.Jain, A. K., Tawari, M., Rathore, L., Sahana, D., Mishra, H., Kumar, S., & Sahu, R. K. (2022). An experience with Goel-Harms C1-C2 fixation for type II odontoid fractures. Journal of Craniovertebral Junction and Spine, 13(2), 175–181. https://doi.org/10.4103/jcvjs.jcvjs_22_22

171.Tam, S. K. P., Bolognese, P. A., Kula, R. W., Brodbelt, A., Foroughi, M., Avshalumov, M., Mugutso, D., & Ruhoy, I. (2022). Safety analysis and complications of condylar screws in a single-surgeon series of 250 occipitocervical fusions. Acta Neurochirurgica, 164(3), 903–911. https://doi.org/10.1007/s00701-021-05039-z

172.Honey, C. (2023). The tenth nerve: A brain surgeon's stories of the patients who changed him. Random House Canada.(Book)

173.Weill Cornell Medicine. (n.d.). Doctors who treat craniocervical junction disorders. Weill Cornell Medicine Neurological Surgery. Retrieved May 8, 2025, from https://neurosurgery.weillcornell.org/condition/craniocervical-junction-disorders/doctors-who-treat-craniocervical-junction-disorders

174.Oliver, B., & Elenwoke, N. (n.d.). Surgical treatment of Chiari malformation. Chiari Surgery. Retrieved May 8, 2025, from https://chiarisurgery.com/

175.National Institute of Neurological Disorders and Stroke [NIHNINDS]. (2024, January 5). ME/CFS Research Roadmap Webinar – Lesser Studied Pathologies [Video]. YouTube. ME/CFS Research Roadmap Webinar - Lesser Studied Pathologies

176.Bobby Jones Chiari & Syringomyelia Foundation. (n.d.). Surgical interventions. Retrieved May 8, 2025, from https://bobbyjonescsf.org/physician-information/surgical-interventions/

177.Gilete, V. (n.d.). Craniocervical instability diagnosis. Dr. Gilete. Retrieved May 8, 2025, from https://drgilete.com/specialties-craniocervical-instability/

178.Bluestein, L. (Host), & Chopra, P. (Guest). (2023, November 2). 77. Neurosurgical insights from Paolo Bolognese, MD and guest cohost Pradeep Chopra, MD [Audio podcast episode]. In The Bendy Bodies Podcast. Bendy Bodies. https://www.bendybodiespodcast.com/77-neurosurgical-insights-from-paolo-bolognese-md-and-guest-cohost-pradeep-chopra-md/

179.Henderson, F. C., Francomano, C. A., Koby, M., Tuchman, K., Adcock, J., & Patel, S. (2019). Cervical medullary syndrome secondary to craniocervical instability and ventral brainstem compression in hereditary hypermobility connective tissue disorders: 5-year follow-up after craniocervical reduction, fusion, and stabilization. Neurosurgical Review, 42(4), 915–936. https://doi.org/10.1007/s10143-018-01070-4

180.Nayyar, N. S. (2024). A case report on symptomatic internal jugular venous compression: Clinical and radiographic improvement with bilateral C1 tubercle resection. Medical Research Archives, 12(5). https://doi.org/10.18103/mra.v12i5.5415

181. Bolognese, P. A. [EDS Awareness]. (2023, October 15). EDS Awareness Dr. Paolo Bolognese presents Chiari I Malformation, EDS, and Craniocervical Instability [Video]. YouTube. https://youtu.be/MsYDA3SXTkg

182. Goel, A. (2016). Central or axial atlantoaxial instability: Expanding understanding of craniovertebral junction. Journal of Craniovertebral Junction and Spine, 7(1), 1–3. https://doi.org/10.4103/0974-8237.176602

183. Bohra, H., Maalouly, J., Chopra, N., Stewart, C., & others. (2024). Halo traction evaluation of craniocervical instability in hereditary connective tissue disorder patients: Case series. Research Square. https://doi.org/10.21203/rs.3.rs-3183687/v1

184. Henderson, F. C., Francomano, C. A., Koby, M., & others. (2019). Cervical medullary syndrome secondary to craniocervical instability and ventral brainstem compression in hereditary hypermobility connective tissue disorders: 5-year follow-up after craniocervical reduction, fusion, and stabilization. Neurosurgical Review, 42(4), 915–936. https://doi.org/10.1007/s10143-018-01070-4

185. Chiari EDS Center. (n.d.). New patients. Chiari EDS Center. Retrieved May 8, 2025, from https://chiarieds.com/new-patients/

186. Health Rising. (2023, October 28). Kaufman & Ruhoy: Craniocervical instability & chronic fatigue syndrome. Health Rising. Retrieved May 8, 2025, from https://www.healthrising.org/blog/2023/10/28/kaufman-ruhoy-craniocervical-instability-chronic-fatigue-syndrome/

187. American College of Surgeons. (1996, September 1). Statement on principles underlying perioperative responsibility. https://www.facs.org/about-acs/statements/principles-underlying-perioperative-responsibility/

188. Chen Q, Brahimaj BC, Khanna R, Kerolus MG, Tan LA, David BT, Fessler RG. Posterior atlantoaxial fusion: a comprehensive review of surgical techniques and relevant vascular anomalies. J Spine Surg. 2020 Mar;6(1):164-180.doi: 10.21037/jss.2020.03.05.. PMID: 32309655; PMCID: PMC7154353.

189. Joaquim AF, Tedeschi H, Chandra PS. Controversies in the surgical management of congenital craniocervical junction disorders - A critical review. Neurol India. 2018 Jul-Aug;66(4):1003-1015. doi: 10.4103/0028-3886.237025. PMID: 30038084.

190. Zileli M, Akıntürk N. Complications of occipitocervical fixation: retrospective review of 128 patients with 5-year mean follow-up. Eur Spine J. 2022 Feb;31(2):311-326. doi: 10.1007/s00586-021-07037-2. Epub 2021 Nov 2. PMID: 34725722.

191. Bobby Jones CSF. (n.d.). Controversial topics. Bobby Jones CSF. Retrieved May 6, 2025, from https://bobbyjonescsf.org/controversial-topics/

192. Duan W, Du Y, Qi T, Jiang B, Wang K, Liu Z, Guan J, Wang X, Wu H, Chen Z, Jian F. The Value and Limitation of Cervical Traction in the Evaluation of the Reducibility of Atlantoaxial Dislocation and Basilar Invagination Using the Intraoperative O-Arm. World Neurosurg. 2019 Dec;132:e324-e332. doi: 10.1016/j.wneu.2019.08.160. Epub 2019 Aug 30. PMID: 31476460.

193. Fehlings, M. G., Ahn, H., Arvin, B., Mroz, T., Brodke, D. S., & Shaffrey, C. I. (2005). Controversies in cervical discectomy and fusion: Practice patterns among Canadian spine surgeons. Spine, 30(16), E443–E449. https://doi.org/10.1097/01.brs.0000173893.67527.37

194. Deyo, R. A., Nachemson, A., & Mirza, S. K. (2004). Spinal-fusion surgery — The case for restraint. The New England Journal of Medicine, 350(7), 722–726. https://doi.org/10.1056/NEJMsb031771

195. Lin, M.-S., Huang, C.-W., Tsou, H.-K., Tzeng, C.-Y., Kao, T.-H., Lin, R.-H., Chen, T.-Y., Li, C.-R., & Lee, C.-Y. (2023). Advances in surgical treatment for atlantoaxial instability focusing on rheumatoid arthritis: Analysis of a series of 67 patients. International Journal of Rheumatic Diseases. https://doi.org/10.1111/1756-185X.14855

196. Resnick, D. K., Shaffrey, C. I., Rhee, J. M., & Patel, A. A. (2021). Cervical fusion for treatment of degenerative conditions: Development of appropriate use criteria. Spine, 46(14), E755–E763. https://doi.org/10.1097/BRS.0000000000003990

197. Park, C., Shaffrey, C. I., Than, K. D., Michalopoulos, G. D., El Sammak, S., Chan, A. K., Bisson, E. F., Sherrod, B. A., Asher, A. L., Coric, D., Potts, E. A., Foley, K. T., Wang, M. Y., Fu, K. M., Virk, M. S., Knightly, J. J., Meyer, S., Park, P., Upadhyaya, C., Shaffrey, M. E., Buchholz, A. L., Tumialán, L. M., Turner, J., Agarwal, N., Chou, D., Chaudhry, N. S., Haid, R. W., Mummaneni, P. V., Bydon, M., & Gottfried, O. N. (2023). What factors influence surgical decision-making in anterior versus posterior surgery for cervical myelopathy? A QOD analysis. Journal of Neurosurgery: Spine, 40(2), 206–215. https://doi.org/10.3171/2023.8.SPINE23194

198. Irwin, Z. N., Hilibrand, A., Gustavel, M., McLain, R., Shaffer, W., Myers, M., Glaser, J., & Hart, R. A. (2005). Variation in surgical decision making for degenerative spinal disorders. Part II: Cervical spine. Spine, 30(19), 2214–2219. https://doi.org/10.1097/01.brs.0000181056.76595.f7

199. UCSF Brain Tumor Center. (n.d.). Neurosurgery inpatient caregiver program. University of California, San Francisco. Retrieved May 6, 2025, from https://braintumorcenter.ucsf.edu/support/caregiver/caregiver-resources/neurosurgery-inpatient-caregiver-program

200. Solace Health. (n.d.). Caregiver support. Retrieved May 6, 2025, from https://www.solace.health/specialty/caregiver-support

201. Mao G, Kopparapu S, Jin Y, Davidar AD, Hersh AM, Weber-Levine C, Theodore N. Craniocervical instability in patients with Ehlers-Danlos syndrome: controversies in diagnosis and management. Spine J. 2022 Dec;22(12):1944-1952. doi: 10.1016/j.spinee.2022.08.008. Epub 2022 Aug 24. PMID: 36028216. https://pubmed.ncbi.nlm.nih.gov/36028216/

Chapter 3

202. Joaquim AF, Schroeder GD, Vaccaro AR. Traumatic Atlanto-Occipital Dislocation-A Comprehensive Analysis of All Case Series Found in the Spinal Trauma Literature. Int J Spine Surg. 2021 Aug;15(4):724-739. doi: 10.14444/8095. Epub 2021 Jul 21. PMID: 34289992; PMCID: PMC8375687.

203. Yang SY, Boniello AJ, Poorman CE, Chang AL, Wang S, Passias PG. A review of the diagnosis and treatment of atlantoaxial dislocations. Global Spine J. 2014 Aug;4(3):197-210. doi: 10.1055/s-0034-1376371. Epub 2014 May 22. PMID: 25083363; PMCID: PMC4111952.

204. Lvov I, Grin A, Talypov A, Smirnov V, Kordonsky A, Barbakadze Z, Abdrafiev R, Krylov V. Efficacy and Safety of Goel-Harms Technique in Upper Cervical Spine Surgery: A Systematic Review and Meta-Analysis. World Neurosurg. 2022 Nov;167:e1169-e1184. doi: 10.1016/j.wneu.2022.09.016. Epub 2022 Sep 8. PMID: 36089281.

205. Hofler RC, Pecoraro N, Jones GA. Outcomes of Surgical Correction of Atlantoaxial Instability in Patients with Down Syndrome: Systematic Review and Meta-Analysis. World Neurosurg. 2019 Jun;126:e125-e135. doi: 10.1016/j.wneu.2019.01.267. Epub 2019 Feb 18. PMID: 30790735.

206. Henderson FC Sr, Schubart JR, Narayanan MV, Tuchman K, Mills SE, Poppe DJ, Koby MB, Rowe PC, Francomano CA. Craniocervical instability in patients with Ehlers-Danlos syndromes: outcomes analysis following occipito-cervical fusion. Neurosurg Rev. 2024 Jan 2;47(1):27. doi: 10.1007/s10143-023-02249-0. PMID: 38163828; PMCID: PMC10758368.

207. Ruhoy Ilene S. , Bolognese Paolo A. , Rosenblum Jared S. , Dass Randall A. , Nayyer Navdeep S. , Wood Jeffrey D. , Biggins John B. Comorbidities and neurosurgical interventions in a cohort with connective tissue disorders Frontiers in Neurology Volume 15 - 2024 2025 https://www.frontiersin.org/journals/neurology/articles/10.3389/fneur.2024.1484504 10.3389/fneur.2024.1484504. ISSN=1664-2295

208. Wang M, Shen J, Tan J, Zhu X, Ma H, Wen Z, Tian Y, Jiang W. Risk factors for cervical instability in rheumatoid arthritis: a meta-analysis. Arch Med Sci. 2024 Mar 5;20(2):375-383. doi: 10.5114/aoms/173494. PMID: 38757018; PMCID: PMC11094836.

209. Grob D, Schütz U, Plötz G. Occipitocervical fusion in patients with rheumatoid arthritis. Clin Orthop Relat Res. 1999 Sep;(366):46-53. PMID: 10627717.https://pubmed.ncbi.nlm.nih.gov/10627717/

210. Schizas C, de Goumoëns P, Fragnière B. Chirurgie de la colonne cervicale rhumatoïde [Rheumatoid arthritis of the cervical spine: surgical management]. Rev Med Suisse Romande. 2004 Sep;124(9):575-8. French. PMID: 15552754.https://pubmed.ncbi.nlm.nih.gov/15552754/

211. Streufert BD, Onyedinma C, Yolcu YU, Ghaith AK, Elder BD, Nassr A, Currier B, Sebastian AS, Bydon M. Rheumatoid Arthritis in Spine Surgery: A Systematic Review and Meta-Analysis. Global Spine J. 2022 Sep;12(7):1583-1595. doi: 10.1177/21925682211057543. Epub 2022 Mar 18. PMID: 35302407; PMCID: PMC9393968.

212. Wang AJ, Huang KT, Smith TR, Lu Y, Chi JH, Groff MW, Zaidi HA. Cervical Spine Osteomyelitis: A Systematic Review of Instrumented Fusion in the Modern Era. World Neurosurg. 2018 Dec;120:e562-e572. doi: 10.1016/j.wneu.2018.08.129. Epub 2018 Aug 28. PMID: 30165226.

213. Sadek AR, Wallage W, Jaiganesh T. Cervical spine tuberculosis causing instability and neurological compromise. JRSM Short Rep. 2011 Jun;2(6):47. doi: 10.1258/shorts.2011.011040. Epub 2011 Jun 6. PMID: 21731817; PMCID: PMC3127497.

214. Konbaz FS, Alessia SI, Al Helal FH, Abalkhail MS, Alamri AJ, Saeed AI et al.: Upper cervical spine instability due to pyogenic infection successfully treated by one stage posterior debridement and stabilization: case report and literature review. J Musculoskelet Surg Res 2021;5:303-11.http://dx.doi.org/10.25259/JMSR_14_2021

215. Ferdinandov D, Yankov D, Bussarsky A. Grisel's syndrome in adults: A case report. Surg Neurol Int. 2021 Jan 13;12:15. doi: 10.25259/SNI_733_2020. PMID: 33500830; PMCID: PMC7827359.

216. Nakai A, Uehara M, Miyaoka Y, Oba H, Ikegami S, Takizawa T, Munakata R, Hatakenaka T, Kamanaka T, Kurogochi D, Fukuzawa T, Takahashi J. A case of adult-onset Grisel's syndrome. Br J Neurosurg. 2024 Dec;38(6):1319-1321. doi: 10.1080/02688697.2022.2061420. Epub 2022 Apr 8. PMID: 35393919.

217. Chua AJK, Tan BWS, Tan TY, Heah HHW. Grisel's Syndrome in an Adult After Endoscopic Nasopharyngectomy. Laryngoscope Investig Otolaryngol. 2019 Aug 13;4(5):504-507. doi: 10.1002/lio2.298. PMID: 31637293; PMCID: PMC6793604.

218. Bocciolini C, Dall'Olio D, Cunsolo E, Cavazzuti PP, Laudadio P. Grisel's syndrome: a rare complication following adenoidectomy. Acta Otorhinolaryngol Ital. 2005 Aug;25(4):245-9. PMID: 16482983; PMCID: PMC2639892.10.25259/JMSR_14_2021

219. Ugur HC, Cağlar S, Unlu A, Erdem A, Kanpolat Y. Infection-related atlantoaxial subluxation in two adults: Grisel syndrome or not? Acta Neurochir (Wien). 2003 Jan;145(1):69-72. doi: 10.1007/s00701-002-0979-5. PMID: 12545265.

220. Barker S, Mujallid R, Bayanzay K. Atlantoaxial Subluxation Secondary to SARS-CoV-2 Infection: A Rare Orthopedic Complication from COVID-19. Am J Case Rep. 2022 Jul 19;23:e936128. doi: 10.12659/AJCR.936128. PMID: 35851056; PMCID: PMC9308481.

221. Al-Hussain OH, Al-Hussain G. Diagnostic Approach and Treatment Options for Pediatric Cases of Grisel's Syndrome Post Otolaryngology Procedure: A Systematic Review. Cureus. 2024 Jan 6;16(1):e51739. doi: 10.7759/cureus.51739. PMID: 38187032; PMCID: PMC10771032.

222. Alan N, Cohen JA, Zhou J, Pease M, Kanter AS, Okonkwo DO, Hamilton DK. Top 50 most-cited articles on craniovertebral junction surgery. J Craniovertebr Junction Spine. 2017 Jan-Mar;8(1):22-32. doi: 10.4103/0974-8237.199883. PMID: 28250633; PMCID: PMC5324355.

223. Gorbacheva A, Pierre C, Gerstmeyer J, Davis DD, Anderson BG, Heffernan T, Jouppi L, Daher Z, Tabesh A, Lockey S, Abdul-Jabbar A, Oskouian R, Chapman JR. Recent Global Trends and Hotspots in Occipitocervical Fusion: A Bibliometric Analysis and Visualization Study. World Neurosurg. 2025 Jan;193:1008-1016. doi: 10.1016/j.wneu.2024.09.128 Epub 2024 Oct 23. PMID: 39366481

224. Henderson FC Sr, Schubart JR, Narayanan MV, Tuchman K, Mills SE, Poppe DJ, Koby MB, Rowe PC, Francomano CA. Craniocervical instability in patients with Ehlers-Danlos syndromes: outcomes analysis following occipito-cervical fusion. Neurosurg Rev. 2024 Jan 2;47(1):27. doi: 10.1007/s10143-023-02249-0. PMID: 38163828; PMCID: PMC10758368.

225. da Silva OT, Ghizoni E, Tedeschi H, Joaquim AF. Role of dynamic computed tomography scans in patients with congenital craniovertebral junction malformations. World J Orthop. 2017 Mar 18;8(3):271-277. doi: 10.5312/wjo.v8.i3.271. PMID: 28361020; PMCID: PMC5359763.

226. Tijanić M, Burić N, Burić K. The Use of Cone Beam CT(CBCT) in Differentiation of True from Mimicking Eagle Syndrome. Int J Environ Res Public Health. 2020 Aug 5;17(16):5654. doi: 10.3390/ijerph17165654. PMID: 32764440; PMCID: PMC7459491.

227. Mahdavi A, Rasti S. Dynamic Flexion-Extension Magnetic Resonance Imaging of the Cervical Spine: An Evolutionary Tool for Diagnosis and Management of Cervical Spondylotic Myelopathy. World Neurosurg. 2024 Apr;184:138-147. doi: 10.1016/j.wneu.2024.01.081. Epub 2024 Jan 20. PMID: 38246532.

228. Yanni DS, Ozgur BM, Louis RG, Shekhtman Y, Iyer RR, Boddapati V, Iyer A, Patel PD, Jani R, Cummock M, Herur-Raman A, Dang P, Goldstein IM, Brant-Zawadzki M, Steineke T, Lenke LG. Real-time navigation guidance with intraoperative CT imaging for pedicle screw placement using an augmented reality head-mounted display: a proof-of-concept study. Neurosurg Focus. 2021 Aug;51(2):E11. doi: 10.3171/2021.5.FOCUS21209. PMID: 34333483.

229. Alqurashi A, Alomar SA, Bakhaidar M, Alfiky M, Baeesa SS. Accuracy of Pedicle Screw Placement Using Intraoperative CT-Guided Navigation and Conventional Fluoroscopy for Lumbar Spondylosis. Cureus. 2021 Aug 25;13(8):e17431. doi: 10.7759/cureus.17431. PMID: 34462711; PMCID: PMC8389880.

230. Kataria R, Mehrotra M, Purohit DK, Gupta A, Rathore M. Prediction of the functional and radiological outcome on the basis of independent factors with special emphasis on the use of 3D printed models in craniovertebral junction surgery. Surg Neurol Int. 2022 Aug 19;13:369. doi: 10.25259/SNI_998_2021. PMID: 36128135; PMCID: PMC9479533.

231. Alemayehu DG, Zhang Z, Tahir E, Gateau D, Zhang DF, Ma X. Preoperative Planning Using 3D Printing Technology in Orthopedic Surgery. Biomed Res Int. 2021 Oct 12;2021:7940242. doi: 10.1155/2021/7940242. PMID: 34676264; PMCID: PMC8526200.

232. Kataria R, Mehrotra M, Purohit DK, Gupta A, Rathore M. Prediction of the functional and radiological outcome on the basis of independent factors with special emphasis on the use of 3D printed models in craniovertebral junction surgery. Surg Neurol Int. 2022 Aug 19;13:369. doi: 10.25259/SNI_998_2021. PMID: 36128135; PMCID: PMC9479533.

233. Alluri RK, Avrumova F, Sivaganesan A, Vaishnav AS, Lebl DR, Qureshi SA. Overview of Robotic Technology in Spine Surgery. HSS J. 2021 Oct;17(3):308-316. doi: 10.1177/15563316211026647. Epub 2021 Jul 1. PMID: 34539272; PMCID: PMC8436343.

234. Lebl DR, Avrumova F, Abjornson C, Cammisa FP. Cervical Spine Navigation and Enabled Robotics: A New Frontier in Minimally Invasive Surgery. HSS J. 2021 Oct;17(3):333-343. doi: 10.1177/15563316211026652. Epub 2021 Jul 1. PMID: 34539275; PMCID: PMC8436338.

235. Elswick CM, Strong MJ, Joseph JR, Saadeh Y, Oppenlander M, Park P. Robotic-Assisted Spinal Surgery: Current Generation Instrumentation and New Applications. Neurosurg Clin N Am. 2020 Jan;31(1):103-110. doi: 10.1016/j.nec.2019.08.012. Epub 2019 Oct 25. PMID: 31739920.

236. Halderman AA, Barnett SL. Endoscopic endonasal approach to the craniovertebral junction. World J Otorhinolaryngol Head Neck Surg. 2022 Mar 14;8(1):16-24. doi: 10.1002/wjo2.8. PMID: 35619929; PMCID: PMC9126158.

237. Morales-Valero SF, Serchi E, Zoli M, Mazzatenta D, Van Gompel JJ. Endoscopic endonasal approach for craniovertebral junction pathology: a review of the literature. Neurosurg Focus. 2015 Apr;38(4):E15. doi: 10.3171/2015.1.FOCUS14831. PMID: 25828491.

238. Innovations in craniovertebral junction training: harnessing the power of mixed reality and head-mounted displays Akshay Ganeshkumar MBBS, Varidh Katiyar MCh, Prachi Singh MBBS, Ravi Sharma MCh, Amol Raheja MCh, Kanwaljeet Garg MCh, Shashwat Mishra MCh, Vivek Tandon MCh, Ajay Garg DM, Franco Servadei MD, and Shashank Sharad Kale MCh Page Range: E13 Volume/ Issue: Volume 56: Issue 1 DOI link: https://doi.org/10.3171/2023.10.FOCUS23613

239. Filimonov A, Zeiger J, Goldrich D, Nayak R, Govindaraj S, Bederson J, Shrivastava R, Iloreta AMC. Virtual reality surgical planning for endoscopic endonasal approaches to the craniovertebral junction. Am J Otolaryngol. 2022 Jan-Feb;43(1):103219. doi: 10.1016/j.amjoto.2021.103219. Epub 2021 Sep 11. PMID: 34536921.

240. Blanco, J.F., Villarón, E.M., Pescador, D. et al. Autologous mesenchymal stromal cells embedded in tricalcium phosphate for posterolateral spinal fusion: results of a prospective phase I/II clinical trial with long-term follow-up. Stem Cell Res Ther 10, 63 (2019). https://doi.org/10.1186/s13287-019-1166-4

241. Hagemann C, Stücker R, Schmitt I, Höller A, Kunkel P. Posterior fusion of the craniocervical junction in the pediatric spine: Wright's translaminar C2 screw technique provides for more safety and effectiveness. Eur Spine J. 2020 May;29(5):970-976. doi: 10.1007/s00586-020-06368-w. Epub 2020 Mar 16. PMID: 32180024.

242. Martínez-Lage, J.F., Alarcón, F., Alfaro, R. et al. Severe spinal cord injury in craniocervical dislocation. Case-based update. Childs Nerv Syst 29, 187–194 (2013). https://doi.org/10.1007/s00381-012-1915-5

243. Upadhyaya M, Jain S, Kire N, Merchant Z, Kundnani V, Patel A. Surgical, clinical, and radiological outcomes of occipitocervical fusion using the plate-screw-rod system with allograft in craniocervical instability. J Craniovertebr Junction Spine. 2019 Oct-Dec;10(4):216-223. doi: 10.4103/jcvjs.JCVJS_87_19. Epub 2020 Jan 23. PMID: 32089614; PMCID: PMC7008657.

244. Choi SH, Lee SG, Park CW, Kim WK, Yoo CJ, Son S. Surgical outcomes and complications after occipito-cervical fusion using the screw-rod system in craniocervical instability. J Korean Neurosurg Soc. 2013 Apr;53(4):223-7. doi: 10.3340/jkns.2013.53.4.223. Epub 2013 Apr 30. PMID: 23826478; PMCID: PMC3698232.

245. Sosa-Nájera A, Tafur-Grandett AA, Ceja-Espinosa A, Huato-Reyes R, Ortega-Espino J. Report of two cases of high cervical injury: an adequate functional result with timely surgical management. Cir Cir. 2023 May 11;92(5):668-673. doi: 10.24875/CIRU.21000719. PMID: 37169363.

246. Goel A, Dhar A, Shah A, Rai S, Bakale N, Vaja T. Revision for Failed Craniovertebral Junction Stabilization: A Report of 30 Treated Cases. World Neurosurg. 2019 Jul;127:e856-e863. doi: 10.1016/j.wneu.2019.03.286. Epub 2019 Apr 5. PMID: 30954741..

247.Cappuccio, M., De Iure, F., Amendola, L. et al. Occipito-cervical fusion in post-traumatic instability of the upper cervical spine and cranio-cervical junction. Eur Spine J 22 (Suppl 6), 900–904 (2013). https://doi.org/10.1007/s00586-013-3015-y

248.Joaquim AF, Osorio JA, Riew KD. Occipitocervical Fixation: General Considerations and Surgical Technique. Global Spine J. 2020 Aug;10(5):647-656. doi: 10.1177/2192568219877878. Epub 2019 Sep 24. PMID: 32677563; PMCID: PMC7359687

249.Richards, O., Saeed, F., Derham, C., & Tyagi, A. (2023). Craniocervical fusion in the paediatric population – case series of 21 patients. British Journal of Neurosurgery, 38(1), 116–121. https://doi.org/10.1080/02688697.2023.2170329

250.Nishikawa M, Bolognese PA, Yamagata T, Naito K, Sakamoto H, Hara M, Ohata K, Goto T. Surgical management of Chiari malformation type i and instability of the craniocervical junction based on its pathogenesis and classification. Neurologia medico-chirurgica. 2022 Sep 15;62(9):400-15.doi: 10.2176/jns-nmc.2022-0078.

251.Nishikawa M, Bolognese PA, Kula RW, Ikuno H, Takami T, Ohata K. Surgical management of Chiari malformations: preliminary results of surgery according to the mechanisms of ptosis of the brainstem and cerebellum. Journal of Neurological Surgery Part B: Skull Base. 2021 Apr;82(02):264-72.doi: 10.2176/jns-nmc.2022-0078

252.Henderson, F. C., Francomano, C. A., Koby, M., Tuchman, K., Adcock, J., & Patel, S. (2018, December 10). Cervical medullary syndrome secondary to craniocervical instability and ventral brainstem compression in hereditary hypermobility connective tissue disorders: 5-year follow-up after craniocervical reduction, fusion, and stabilization. Neurosurgical Review. https://doi.org/10.1007/s10143-018-01070-4

253.Tam, Sharon & Bolognese, Paolo & Kula, Roger & Brodbelt, Andrew & Foroughi, Mansoor & Avshalumov, Marat & Mugutso, Denmark & Ruhoy, Ilene. (2022). Safety analysis and complications of condylar screws in a single-surgeon series of 250 occipitocervical fusions. Acta Neurochirurgica. 164. 10.1007/s00701-021-05039-z.

254.Chae, J. K., Marianayagam, N. J., Hussain, I., Cruz, A., Baaj, A. A., Härtl, R., & Greenfield, J. P. New York (2021). Predicting clinical outcomes using morphometric changes in adults with complex Chiari malformation undergoing occipitocervical fusion with or without ventral decompression: patient series. Journal of Neurosurgery: Case Lessons, 2(22), CASE21364. https://doi.org/10.3171/CASE21364

Obtain 2nd Radiology Opinions at:

SPINEANDBRAINADVOCATE.COM

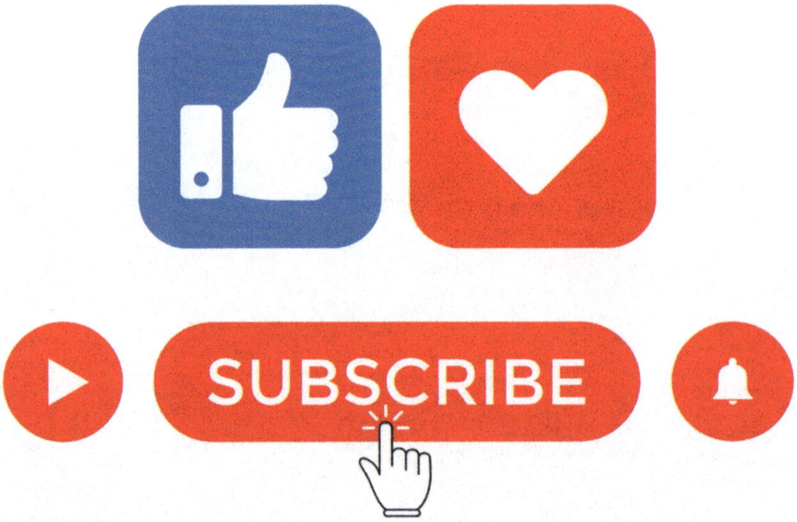

https://www.youtube.com/@spineandbrainadvocate

Facebook: Spine & Brain Advocate

Website: spineandbrainadvocate.com

Made in United States
Orlando, FL
04 November 2026

90200948R00109